0 641 503 00 65

KU-310-018

Interviewing and Patient Care

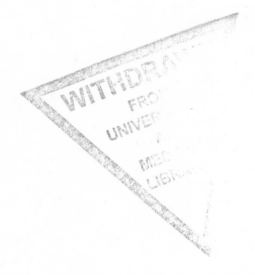

WITHDRAWN
FROM
UNIVER
MED
LIBRA

Interviewing and Patient Care

FOURTH EDITION

ALLEN J. ENELOW, M.D.
University of Southern California

DOUGLAS L. FORDE, M.D.
University of Southern California

KENNETH BRUMMEL-SMITH, M.D.
Oregon Health Sciences University

New York   Oxford
OXFORD UNIVERSITY PRESS
1996

610.696   R726.5
       ene

Oxford University Press

Oxford   New York
Athens   Auckland   Bangkok   Bombay
Calcutta   Cape Town   Dar es Salaam   Delhi
Florence   Hong Kong   Istanbul   Karachi
Kuala Lumpur   Madras   Madrid   Melbourne
Mexico City   Nairobi   Paris   Singapore
Taipei   Tokyo   Toronto

and associated companies in
Berlin   Ibadan

Copyright © 1972, 1979, 1986, 1996 by Oxford University Press, Inc.

Published by Oxford University Press, Inc.,
198 Madison Avenue, New York, New York 10016

All rights reserved. No part of this publication may be reproduced,
stored in a retrieval system, or transmitted, in any form or by any means,
electronic, mechanical, photocopying, recording, or otherwise,
without the prior permission of Oxford University Press.

Library of Congress Cataloging-in-Publication Data
Enelow, Allen J. (Allen Jay), 1922–
Interviewing and patient care.—4th ed. / Allen J. Enelow.
Douglas L. Forde, Kenneth Brummel-Smith.
p. cm. Includes bibliographical references and index.
ISBN 0-19-506443-7 (cloth).—ISBN 0-19-506444-5 (paper)
1. Medical history taking. 2. Physician and patient. I. Forde, Douglas L.
II. Brummel-Smith, Kenneth. III. Title.
[DNLM: 1. Medical History Taking—methods. 2. Physician Patient Relations.
WB 290 E56i 1996]
RC65.E54   1996
610.69′6—dc20
DNLM/DLC
for Library of Congress 95-50440

B WC

9 8 7 6 5 4 3 2 1

Printed in the United States of America
on acid-free paper

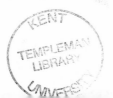
KENT
TEMPLEMAN
LIBRARY
UNIVE...

641503

PREFACE

Twenty-four years have passed since the first edition of this book appeared. Significant changes have occurred in health care during that time. Many of these changes have had the effect of curtailing the time available to clinicians for interviewing. The demands made on physicians and other health professionals in this era of managed care and economic stringency make it increasingly difficult to keep a patient-centered focus in interviews. There is a real danger of losing sight of the human side of health care as physicians are tempted to respond to time constraints with more focused questions misguidedly aimed at efficiency in data-gathering, at the expense of establishing a helping relationship.

Effective interviewing is the key to inspiring the all-important feeling of trust and confidence in the clinician that is most likely to lead to the patient's following treatment recommendations, increasing the likelihood of a positive outcome. This is best accomplished with an open-ended style of interviewing and data-gathering that is the central theme of this book. Also, to be able to provide the psychologic support that is so important to patients within the more limited time available to the clinical interviewer nowadays, it is even more important now than previously to utilize the principles that we have described in this book.

Chapter 1 sets the tone for the fourth edition. The change in emphasis with this edition is in the direction of anchoring it more firmly in the everyday practice of medicine. Chapter 2 presents several techniques that make for a patient-centered interview. When these become familiar and easy to apply, they can be carried over into every aspect of patient care, as discussed in subsequent chapters.

Chapter 3 contains new material not represented in previous editions on the components of a complete medical history. Chapter 4 also contains new information on interviewing patients from other cultures and other countries of origin, the use of interpreters, and the special considerations in interviewing the mildly cognitively impaired patient, the blind patient, and the hearing-impaired as well as interviews in special care units.

Chapter 5 provides fresh material on the impact of the patient's appearance and behavior on the physician and how this affects the care given. There is an entirely new chapter on interviewing children and their parents by a guest author, Karen Brummel-Smith, M.D. The chapters on interviewing families and on interviewing the older adult were revised and updated from the third edition. Another new chapter, 9, on interviewing in continuing care replaces the chapter on that topic in the third edition. Finally, the book ends with a new chapter by a guest author, Geoffrey Gordon, M.D., on ethical issues and end-of-life-decision-making.

The contributions of many persons have helped to shape this fourth edition of *Interviewing and Patient Care*. The earlier editions were co-authored by Scott Swisher, M.D. whose ideas and contributions are preserved in this edition. Medical students at Michigan State University in the early 1970s and since that time at the University of Southern California have used these concepts and provided critiques of the material in this and previous editions. The initial contributions of Leta McKinney Adler, Ph.D. and Murray Wexler, Ph.D. are still reflected in this edition. The authors also wish to acknowledge the help of Mary Rau and Debbie Fazio, who typed many drafts of every chapter.

Santa Barbara, CA   A. J. E.
January 1996

CONTENTS

Interviewing and Patient Care

1

THE INTERVIEW IN CLINICAL MEDICINE

KEY POINTS

1. The medical interview is concerned with both aspects of the patient's story, the biological and the psychosocial.
2. Diagnoses are based chiefly on the interview.
3. Listening carefully, skillful interviewing, and empathy result in a more effective doctor-patient relationship.

Diagnosis and treatment in medicine begin with the interview. Skillful interviewing is the clinician's most powerful tool in establishing the diagnosis. It is essential to the patient's following treatment recommendations, and is at the heart of the doctor-patient relationship.

A study of the relative contributions of the history, physical examination, and laboratory investigations to establishing medical diagnoses concluded that in 76% of patients the interview led to the diagnosis.[1] Other studies have shown that skilled interviewing results in more accurate and complete diagnoses.[2]

Clinicians are likely to regard the term "medical interview" as synonymous with what is called history-taking. But medical interviewing is more than just history-taking. It is the process whereby the interviewer seeks to understand all the factors—biological, psychological, and social— that play a role in the patient's becoming ill and that will affect his getting well.

TABLE 1.1. Requirements for Developing
Effective Interviewing Skills

---

1. Refine your listening skills
2. Practice interviewing techniques
3. Establish rapport with the patient

While diagnosis is the first step in the patient-physician encounter, explaining what is wrong, recommending treatment, and obtaining a commitment to work together also require good interviewing and different skills than those used in gathering the medical and psychosocial data. In telling the patient what is wrong, the clinician should use words that will be understood and not unduly frightening. The physician must consider the patient's expectations and desires, elicit the patient's own ideas about the cause of the illness, and respect those belief systems that may differ from his own. Educating the patient about his illness and treatment entails a two-way discussion that is quite different from the patient-centered format of the diagnostic interview. These various aspects of the medical interview are all discussed in this book.

The interview is the basis for the positive side of health care that is often sought in vain by patients. Patients desire a special relationship with their doctor. This relationship is an important aspect of helping a sick person get better.[3] The physician does not limit his help to the removal of physical pain and other symptoms but seeks to produce a state of comfort and feeling of well-being in the patient. Studies have shown that patients' satisfaction with their medical care relates more to doctors' consideration of the psychosocial than the biological features of illness.[4]

To become a good interviewer, the student-physician and clinician alike must learn to listen, learn effective interviewing techniques, and discover how to establish rapport with the patient (Table 1.1).

LISTENING TO THE PATIENT

"Listen to the patient, he is telling you the diagnosis" was a dictum of the famed nineteenth century physician, Sir William Osler.[5] By listening attentively to that story, the physician obtains information needed for a diagnosis. This includes the milieu in which the illness takes place—home, workplace, or even the streets—the people in the patient's life, and significant recent events. The clinician listens to the words, the feeling behind them, and their context. The sociocultural story that accompanies the biomedical concerns has been termed the "voice of the life world."[6] As Mishler suggests, too often only the "voice of medicine" is heard, and it stresses the patient's biological symptoms. To understand the illness and the person with that illness, it is necessary to listen to both voices. In so doing, the clinician may learn the patient's real reasons for the visit, as well as his or her beliefs about the illness. Often of equal importance is information about the effects of the illness on the patient's life.

Some of those entering the health professions are instinctively good listeners. Their peers seek them out to tell them their troubles and ask for advice. Other students may not initially possess good listening skills, but they can learn. Listening to a patient, however, is different from listening to a friend or acquaintance. It is also different from television interviews where the interviewer asks a series of questions. Professional listening allows the patient to tell his own story aided by the interviewing techniques described in Chapter 2. In this type of interview questions are withheld early in the interview and the patient is encouraged to speak without interruption. Relieved of the need to ask questions, the interviewer can concentrate on listening carefully to the patient's story rather than on mentally framing the next question while the patient is relating his history.

The stories patients tell about their illnesses and their lives are almost always interesting. Their stories are made of medical facts entwined with personal problems, each affecting the other.[7] Some patients are easier to listen to than others. They talk of their symptoms and their lives with animation, gestures, and even humor. Some are articulate and describe their illnesses with great clarity. Others make listening more difficult. They can be angry or sad. They may speak in a monotonous tone with an unemotional manner, or they may be difficult to follow. Many patients can give only vague descriptions of their illnesses and may be similarly limited in talking about their lives.

Understanding patients' symptoms can be difficult because of differences in the way they describe them. Pain, for example may be described by one patient as excruciatingly severe and by another as only mildly uncomfortable. This is not only due to differences in pain thresholds but also reflects personal histories, cultural backgrounds, and psychological makeup. A patient's age and personal history is likely to be very different from that of the interviewer. The 23-year-old medical student may interview a 15-year-old Hispanic gang member or a 75-year-old college professor. Patients seen in university hospitals today come from many different cultures. They may have beliefs about illness that are radically different from those of the student-physician. Their accounts will be greatly influenced by their own emotional state. Accordingly, knowing the symptoms of a given disease is not sufficient for accurate diagnosis and effective treatment. It is necessary to know the patient as a person, which requires effective interviewing.

Despite its importance, being a good listener is not enough. Interviewing successfully requires learning the art of obtaining a full and accurate medical history, as well as a better understanding of the patient's personal life.

THE TECHNIQUE OF INTERVIEWING

The interviewing techniques described in this book are patient centered. In the patient-centered interview, the patient takes the lead in telling the story of his illness, his ideas regarding its cause, his expectations in coming to the doctor, and his emotional response to the illness. Unlike a physician-centered interview in which the patient's history is elicited by asking a series of questions, the patient-centered interview facilitates the patient's telling his story without interruption until later in the interview when it is necessary to obtain more specific information. Such a story is free of the bias that can result when the physician poses questions that may limit the patient's freedom to respond. It is more accurate because it is generated by the patient. In a physician-centered interview questions asked are usually biomedical in nature as the physician constructs a clinical history from the patient's symptoms. Left on his own, however, the patient will probably describe elements of his personal story along with the medical complaints. Information thus obtained is more likely to be valid and can lead to a better outcome.

Later in the interview, as will be described in Chapter 3, the clinician can become more directive to clarify issues raised earlier. Discussing recommendations and providing patient education includes both patient-centered and physician-centered techniques. A real dialogue takes place as the doctor and patient talk about treatment plans and follow-up visits. Even then, however, the principles employed in a patient-centered encounter are important because they allow the patient to discuss issues about which he was reticent at the beginning of the interview.

A patient-centered interview also promotes the interviewer's expression of empathy for the patient. Empathy develops as the student clinician begins to understand the patient's feelings and the fear and worry that accompany most illnesses.[8] Together with empathic feelings, the clinician will usually feel a sense of contact with the patient and a change in the level of communication.

THE DOCTOR-PATIENT RELATIONSHIP

Most patients want a strong, caring doctor-patient relationship. A good interview promotes such a relationship. Health status and diagnoses change, treatment regimens are modified, but a satisfying professional relationship remains of value to doctor and patient alike. Reiser and Schroder[3] have written, "Repeatedly, physicians feel the power of something intangible, yet unmistakable, in the nature of the doctor-patient relationship that helps a sick person get better. It is hard to overestimate the potency and curative potential of this very unique and special relationship. For all our technical advances, this relationship remains one of medicine's most powerful therapeutic tools."

The student physician who is just learning to interview often feels something intangible between himself and the patient even before he has acquired much knowledge of clinical medicine. It usually happens when the student has been touched by the patient's story and has been

TABLE 1.2. Establishing Rapport

1. Greet the patient warmly
2. Maintain attentive eye contact
3. Use empathic remarks
4. Touch the patient appropriately
5. Discuss personal issues
6. Summarize the encounter sensitively

able to respond with an empathic remark or a show of feeling such as a touch on the patient's hand. It almost always occurs when the patient is discussing personal or psychosocial issues. It rarely happens during the telling of the biomedical history. Sometimes the patient will say he has been able to talk to the student about sensitive issues that he has not been able to discuss with his "doctors." There are, of course, other factors in establishing rapport with the patient (Table 1.2). The manner in which the patient is greeted at the beginning of the interview is important, as is the final summing up or closure at its end. The thoroughness and completeness of the interview, the sensitivity in performing the physical examination, and the skill in discussing the results of the encounter and outlining treatment are all related to the success of the patient-doctor relationship. When the physician recognizes the patient's expectations and wishes for the relationship, the patient's satisfaction with it is increased.[9]

CHANGES IN HEALTH CARE

We have entered an era of change in the traditional doctor-patient relationship. Managed care with much more control by third parties has led to limitation of the amount of time the physician can spend with many, if not most, patients. In many cases, the physician may be unable to devote more than 15 minutes to each patient. Traditionally, physicians have spent up to an hour in carrying out the initial interview, performing the physical examination, and discussing the findings and proposed treatment. The principles of interviewing described in this book are best applied in an unhurried context. For the beginning student interviewer, this is still the best way to learn good interviewing style. Only when one is fully conversant with the ideal interviewing technique and has learned to use it well can he or she modify it successfully to fit time limitations. Then one can achieve knowledge of "the person with the disease, the impact of the disease on the person, the way personal characteristics modify disease presentation, and the family and the community the patient comes from."[10]

CONCLUSION

It has been suggested that poor communication between doctor and patient is at the root of the public's discontent with the medical profession. Good communication is furthered by the principles discussed above: listening well, using patient-centered interviewing techniques, and establishing rapport with the patient. Feelings of confidence and trust are most likely to develop as a result of the physician's ability to meet these goals.

Learning to interview is the central theme of this book. A model for helping the patient to tell his or her story is described. The student clinician can use this model as a guide. Chapter 2 addresses the techniques used in a patient-centered interview. In Chapter 3, the components of a complete medical history are discussed in detail, including the chief complaints, present history, past history, and the environmental factors important in causing disease. Chapter 4 is devoted to interviewing under special circumstances, the non-English speaking patient, the patient from a different culture, the mildly cognitively impaired patient, and a description of a mental status examination. This chapter includes the blind patient as well as the hearing-impaired patient and concludes with interviews in the Emergency Room and the Intensive Care Unit. Emotional responses to patients and to illness are described in Chapter 5. This addresses the impact of the patient on the doctor and how it affects the care received. The special challenges of interviewing children and their parents are explored in Chapter 6. Often patients seen in hospital settings are visited by their families. These situations provide an ideal opportunity to interview the family, which is discussed in Chapter 7. As the number of older persons has increased, their care has created new concerns that are addressed in Chapter 8. These include a short mental status examination, medications, and nutrition. The very important subject of continuing care by the primary care physician is considered in Chapter 9. In this chapter, we discuss reasons why patients see doctors, their expectations and desires, how to open and close an interview, and how illness attributions affect the description of their symptoms. Finally, in Chapter 10 ethical issues and end-of-life decision making are covered.

REFERENCES

1. Burack, R. C., and R. Carpenter, "The Predictive Value of the Presenting Complaint," *The Journal of Family Practice*, 16:749–754, 1983.
2. Peterson, M. C., J. H. Holbrook, M. D. Von Hales, et al., "Contributions of the History, Physical Examination, and Laboratory Investigation in Making Medical Diagnoses," *Western Journal of Medicine*, 156:163–165, 1992.
3. Reiser, D. E., A. K. Schroder, *Patient Interviewing; The Human Dimension*. Baltimore/London: Williams and Wilkins, Chapter 6, 1980.
4. Kravitz, R. L., D. W. Cope, V. Bhrany, et al., "Internal Medicine Patient's Expectations for Care during Office Visits," *Journal of General Internal Medicine*, 9:75–81, 1994.
5. Osler, W., "The Master-word in Medicine," *In Aequanimitas, with other Addresses to Medical Students, Nurses, and Practitioners of Medicine*. Philadelphia: Blakiston, 1904.
6. Mishler, E. G., *The Discourse of Medicine*, Norwood, New Jersey: Ablex Publishing Corporation, 1984.
7. Donnelly, W. J., "Righting the Medical Record: Transforming Chronicle into Story," *Journal of the American Medical Association*, 260,6: 823–825, 1988.
8. Bellet, P. S. and M. J. Maloney, "The Importance of Empathy as an Interviewing Skill in Medicine," *Journal of the American Medical Association*, 266d:1831–1832, 1991.

9. Uhlmann, R. F., W. B. Carter, and T. Inui, "Fulfillment of Patient Requests in a General Medicine Clinic," *American Journal of Public Health*, 74:257–258, 1984.

10. Eisenberg, L., "Medicine—Molecular, Monetary, or More than Both," *Journal of the American Medical Association*, 274:331–334, 1995.

2

BASIC INTERVIEWING

KEY POINTS

1. Open-ended interviewing encourages communication and provides the most useful information.
2. Begin with broad questions and save directive, focused questions for the later part of the interview.
3. Facilitate communication by manner, gesture, or words.
4. Confrontation can reduce tension and provide additional useful information if done supportively.
5. Communication goes on whether or not the clinician or patient is talking.

Sooner or later the beginning medical student must face his or her first patient with a medical illness. This is often frightening. It can inspire feelings of inadequacy and lead to experiences like the following:

The patient, a 40-year-old man, is sitting up in bed. He is clearly jaundiced. The student has attended some initial seminars in which interviewing was discussed and role playing was done, but this is his first real patient.

STUDENT: What kind of problems are you having?
PATIENT: I have fluid on my body. I have liver problems and kidney

problems. I'm short of breath right now—why I don't know. Basically my problem is my liver and my kidney. (*Pause.*)

Patient looks at student clearly waiting for acknowledgement or some response. The student remains silent.

PATIENT: What else do you want?
STUDENT: Tell me about your problem with your liver.
PATIENT: My liver is deteriorating. It doesn't function. I'm tired and I'm anemic.

The patient pauses once again, looking inquiringly at the student. There is still no comment from the student.

PATIENT: That's about all I can tell you. (*The patient pauses again.*)
STUDENT: Can you tell me about the fluid?
PATIENT: There's not much more to say. It's cut and dried. Others are worse than I am.

At this point the patient's eyes and facial expression went blank.

This is a description of an actual encounter during an early Introduction to Clinical Medicine exercise. The student felt helpless. He knew there was much more to be learned but had no idea about how to get the patient's story.

The purpose of this chapter is to describe an interview model and interviewing techniques that will help beginning students learn the essential art of the interview.

PURPOSE OF THE INTERVIEW

Learning to interview does not require a knowledge of medicine. The interview's function is to elicit the story of the patient's medical and psychological or social problems. Learning to interview is actually learning to help the patient tell that story. A large part of medicine is learned at the bedside or in the clinic listening to patients as they tell the story of their symptoms, the impact these have had on their lives, and their emotional response to them.

The purpose of the interview is to get the information needed to establish a working hypothesis about the nature of the patient's problems. This is the first and most important step in arriving at a diagnosis. The interview provides the data from which the clinician can make a tentative diagnosis. It will be followed by a physical examination and usually by laboratory and other studies to confirm that tentative diagnosis. But diagnosis is not the sole function of the interview. Of equal if not greater importance is that it is the first step in forming a therapeutic relationship with the patient.

THE INTERVIEW MODEL

The interview style that has come to be generally accepted as optimal is known as open-ended interviewing. Initially described as the most desirable approach to psychiatric interviewing in 1954,[1] it was modified and adapted to medical interviewing over the next two decades.

There are four general characteristics of this style of interviewing. First, the interview should be carried out in an atmosphere that encourages spontaneous behavior on the part of the patient. Second, the interviewer's behavior should encourage communication. Third, the interviewer should give attention to the patient's nonverbal behavior, or body language, as well as his story. Fourth, the interviewer should begin with questions of a broad sort—open-ended questions—that encourage the patient to tell his story, saving directive or highly focused questions for the later part of the interview.[2] It has been shown that specific questions that are very directive, calling for specific information at the beginning of an interview, interrupt the flow of information from the patient and restrict the range of information the patient will provide.[3]

In summary, the interview model is guided by the principle of exerting the least amount of control consistent with encouraging spontaneous reporting. If it is necessary to use more control to get information, by asking specific questions, this should be done later in the interview.

THE INTERVIEW SETTING

An atmosphere that encourages spontaneous behavior has both physical and emotional attributes. Comfort and privacy should be provided whenever possible. The interviewer should arrange for the fewest possible interruptions.

The private physician conducts most extensive medical interviews in his office, his most congenial environment. This is where he feels most at home and where, consequently, the doctor's most spontaneous behavior is likely to occur. Both the doctor's and the patient's behavior will be influenced by the way the office is used. Both can communicate more freely if the setting of the interview is a quiet consulting room, with reasonably comfortable furniture, and if there are no interruptions. While it is perhaps easiest to secure the conditions for a successful interview in the physician's office, it does not necessarily follow that these conditions will exist. Many physicians permit the telephone and office personnel to interrupt their interviews, do not allow sufficient time for the interview, or narrowly limit the topics discussed. Some physicians make a practice of conducting interviews in their examining rooms, where the patient is partially clothed or under a drape sheet on the examining table. The patient rarely feels at ease under such circumstances and is likely to feel both powerless and self-estranged. The social distance between the doctor and the patient is likely to be increased. Docility, obedience, embarrassment, and efforts to please the physician are likely consequences that will reduce the amount of information from the patient.

The student who is learning to interview does not usually have the advantage of choosing the setting for an interview. Most such interviews in teaching hospitals take place at the bedside, or in clinics. While these are not ideal settings, much can be done to make them more conducive to good communication.

The immediate situation in a hospital is most likely to be unfavorable for an effective interview. The patient is more often than not in a ward or shared room, and hospital personnel or visitors may interrupt the interview. The patient is usually in bed, while the interviewer is clothed and mobile. In this situation, some interviewers stand at the foot of the bed, some at the side of the bed, and some sit on or near the bed while talking to the patient. In each case, the effect on the interview varies. The physical distance from the patient has an effect on the emotional distance; they vary directly with each other. Also, standing over a bed patient suggests that you will not remain long enough for him to tell you very much.

To create a more supportive setting, the interviewer should sit next to the bed—close enough to touch the patient—draw the curtain around the bed in a shared room, and turn his back on others in the hospital room if there is no curtain, thus becoming a barrier between the patient and extraneous persons and objects. Maintaining eye contact makes the interview feel even more private.

Close attention to the patient with its implication of clear interest on the part of the interviewer encourages spontaneous behavior and helps the patient tell his story.

INTRODUCING YOURSELF TO THE PATIENT

Before beginning the interview, the student physician greets the patient. This often poses a problem to the beginning student. How to introduce oneself and how to address the patient become immediate concerns to the student.

Although students usually know the first and last names of the patient and are accustomed to addressing their peers by the first name, this informal social behavior is usually not appropriate when addressing patients. While patients of approximately the same age and sex as the interviewer may sometimes be addressed by the first name, young married women usually prefer being addressed by the married name, particularly by an interviewer of the opposite sex. Patients of different racial or ethnic backgrounds than the interviewer may have strong feelings about how they are addresssed. In any case, patients should be addressed respectfully using the prefix Mr., Ms., or Mrs. (or occasionally Dr.) and the last name. It is the patient's option to suggest use of the first name to the interviewer. In the case of women, if you're uncertain about whether to call the patient Mrs., Miss, or Ms., simply inquire, "How would you like to be addressed?"

It is a good idea to use the patient's name throughout the interview at appropriate points. Patients are pleased when clinicians take the trouble to learn their name. It helps to establish rapport. It is also helpful to the younger student struggling with his or her identity to use the patient's name from time to time, thus defining the exchange as a professional interview. It also reminds the student that the patient is a person and not just a "case."

Introducing oneself as a student physician is usually sufficient, and it is not necessary to add, "I'm just a first-year student," or something similar. This is more of a concern for the student than for the patient. Most patients are happy to be able to tell their story and often thank the student for having taken the time to hear the whole story.

BASIC INTERVIEWING TECHNIQUES

Opening the Interview

The first step in establishing good communication in an initial interview is explaining why you are there. A physician who is about to perform a consultation will usually give his name, area of expertise, and the reason for the interview. For example, he might say, "I'm Dr. Smith. I'm a neurologist. I've been asked by your doctor to examine you." The role of the student is not so clearly defined. A good opening would be, "I'm Mary Jones. I'm a student doctor. I'd like to talk to you to find out why you are here in the hospital and what happened to bring you to this point in your life," or some variation on this opening, depending on your role (intern, resident, student nurse, etc.) and whether you are only going to interview, or will also perform a physical examination.

It is not necessary for the student to explain that he is learning to interview or that his activities are part of his training. Such explanations only confuse the patient. They are self-effacing, apologetic comments whose purpose is to alleviate the student's anxiety. It is also an error to say to the patient, "Tell me a little bit about your problems," as some anxious students do in their concern that they might be told more than they are prepared to hear. This may be interpreted by the patient as the student's desire not to hear too much.

Having established your role and purpose, your next step is to find out the patient's reason for being in the hospital or clinic. This is sometimes called "the chief complaint" and is so labeled in one form of standard history write-up. It is not a good idea to make the chief complaint the focus of your interest in beginning the interview. This can lead to asking to many questions too early. The chief complaint will be discussed more completely in Chapter 3.

An open-ended question such as, "What kind of difficulties are you having?" says to the patient, "I am interested in anything that is of concern to you." Variations on this opening are: "Can you tell me about your problems?" Or, "Please tell me about the problems or symptoms that led to your coming here."

Some patients have difficulty opening up to a stranger, whether doctor, nurse, or student. Such a patient may reply with very few words, such as, "Well, I've been having a lot of headaches," and then fall silent. The clinician may then make the mistake of asking very specific questions about the complaint. It is best to remain open-ended, instead, by saying, "Can you tell me more about that?"

Even when the patient seems to have responded fully and has said a great deal about one or more symptoms, it is sometimes a good idea to ask, "Anything else?" It is not unusual for the most troublesome or frightening problem or symptom to emerge at that time, usually something that worries the patient deeply or about which he feels shame, guilt, or fear. On the other hand, if the patient has described his symptoms in detail with a great deal of feeling, it is best to comment on that. While the patient is talking, it is best to remain silent, i.e., not exercise authority to control the interview. We will say more about the uses of silence later in this chapter.

Facilitation

Encouraging communication by manner, gesture, or words that do not specify the kind of information sought is called facilitation. It encourages the patient to speak freely, to voice his or her concerns and problems without interruption or distraction. It exerts a low degree of control. The interviewer's silence (letting the patient talk) and facilitation tend to go hand in hand. An interested, attentive manner is, of course, facilitating. Any change of facial expression or posture that displays greater interest or attention is a facilitation. A common mode of faciliation is a nod of the head, conveying, "I'm listening," "I understand what you're saying," or, "Go on." This message is encouraging to the patient but can be overused. Inexperienced interviewers frequently relieve their own tension during the interview with what might be called the "head-nodding syndrome." The interviewer should also take pains not to nod his head for facilitating purposes when the patient has been expressing a strong opinion. In such instances, his action may be mistaken for approval or agreement. A similar message is conveyed to the patient with an occasional, "Mmm-mmm," or by postural shifts toward the patient or into a position of greater alertness. The interviewer may also interject short words or phrases such as, "yes," or, "I see," without interrupting the flow of the patient's narrative. Another type of message that is facilitating is the action that conveys, "I don't understand." This may be non-verbal, such as a puzzled look, or a verbal statement of confusion such as, "I don't follow you," or, "I'm sorry, but I don't understand." In short, the clinician's interest in following the patient's account closely is facilitating, encouraging the patient to open up and describe his problems.

When a patient has stopped discussing a topic and falls silent, the interviewer may encourage the patient to continue (after a brief silence to permit the patient to resume spontaneously) by repeating his last few words. This may be done with the inflection of a question or merely as a repetition. For example, either "the last few days" or "the last few days?" will invite the patient to continue. Another verbal facilitation is a brief summary of what the patient has been saying. This indicates that you have understood him and are interested in further information. A brief summarizing remark will usually encourage the patient to continue, without explicitly directing him to do so or specifying what subject he should discuss.

CLINICIAN: What kind of difficulties have you been having?

PATIENT: It's my back.

CLINICIAN: Your back?

PATIENT: Yes. I have pain.

CLINICIAN: Can you tell me more about that?

PATIENT: It hurts all the time. Sometimes the pain goes down my leg, too. It keeps me up at night. And I'm cranky. Any little thing upsets me. It's gotten so my children are afraid of me.

CLINICIAN: What problems are you having?

PATIENT: I feel tired all the time. I don't seem to have any energy. I just want to lie around and do nothing. Everything's an effort.

CLINICIAN: Everything's an effort?

PATIENT: I used to be very active. Full of energy. For the last several months it's been like this.

CLINICIAN: What have the last several months been like?

PATIENT: Well, it started kind of gradually. I noticed that I'd come home from work feeling really tired and I didn't want to do anything. Then I started getting irritable. I wanted to sleep all the time. It just kept getting worse. I started losing weight. I just worked less and less. I couldn't get started. Then my boss said I wasn't doing my job like I used to and I ought to see a doctor.

In the example of the medical student's first interview with which the chapter began, the patient responded to the open-ended question with a summary of his physical problems and then stopped talking. This is quite common. In such instances the patient usually pauses because he is waiting for some acknowledgment from the interviewer either that he has been heard and understood or that he is responding appropriately to the ambiguity of the open-ended question. In this situation, there are several things that the interviewer can do to facilitate communication. One is to recapitulate what the patient has just said while looking at him or her inquiringly. In the brief interchange described at the beginning of this chapter, the student might have said, "You're tried and anemic?" or simply, "Tell me more about that."

Facilitation can also be used to return the patient to a topic previously introduced but not elaborated. This is done by referring to a phrase previously used by the patient, thus indicating that the matter is of interest to the clinician. For example, in the course of describing episodes of chest pain on exertion, the patient mentioned, as though in passing, that he had had shortness of breath on one occasion. After the patient has completed his description, the physician can then say, "You mentioned shortness of breath on one occasion," or, "You mentioned shortness of breath. Tell me about it."

Facilitation promotes communication by suggesting to the patient that the doctor is interested in what he is saying and is encouraging him to continue. It may also prompt the patient to explain or to expand on something he has said. A good interviewer with a normally communicative patient should be able to gain much information by attentive silence and facilitation. When the clinician senses that the patient is not speaking freely and clearly, however, he or she should consider calling attention to the patient's behavior, or to some aspect of it (Table 2.1).

Silence

When a patient falls silent, the interviewer should consider being silent himself for at least a brief time. This is very difficult for the inexperienced interviewer. Ordinarily the patient will soon feel free to resume his account. That the clinician is not speaking does not mean he or she is not communicating. Facial expression, posture, and movements all tell the patient something about the interviewer's response to his account and to him as a person. An attentive facial expression and

TABLE 2.1. Facilitating Techniques

Behavioral	Verbal
Attentive silence	Encouraging remarks:
Nod	"Yes"
Lean forward	"I see"
Facial expression of interest	"Go on"
Look of puzzlement	"Can you tell me more about that?"
	"Anything else?"
	Repeat last few words
	Brief summary

posture tell the patient nonverbally that he has an interested listener. It is a good idea to look at the patient but not stare continuously into the patient's eyes. Looking distracted, fidgeting, slumping in an attitude of fatigue, looking away from the patient, and examining the chart all indicate that the interviewer's attention is not fully focused on the patient. This nonverbal message will inhibit the patient considerably.

Thus, while the patient is communicating freely about important matters, the doctor's behavior of choice is an interested, attentive, and relaxed silence. Whether to remain silent or to speak when the patient falls silent is a choice that requires the skill that comes with experience. During an interview a silence of only a few seconds may seem interminably long and can be quite uncomfortable for the inexperienced interviewer. The busy practitioner is also likely to tolerate silences poorly because of schedule-consciousness. A common response of both beginning and busy practitioners is to search quickly for a question or remark to keep the conversation going. But one can learn to tolerate silences through practice. This is a worthwhile exercise, for there are times in the interview when it is very useful for the clinician to maintain his silence after the patient has stopped speaking.

One of these times is when the patient has stopped speaking in order to clarify his thoughts, to recollect facts, or to find a way of adequately expressing something. The patient may explain such silences with remarks like, "Let me think a minute," or, "How can I say that better?" This kind of thoughtful silence is rarely accompanied by signs of increased tension. The perceptive interviewer can usually recognize this situation and wait for the patient to continue. An interruption may make it more difficult for the patient to express himself clearly.

Another situation requiring a decision either to remain silent or to say something occurs when the patient appears to have said all he wants to say and has come to a natural pause. The pause may be signaled by a remark and by the patient's demeanor, indicating that he has finished and is waiting to hear from you. The best choice at this juncture depends on a number of circumstances.

First, the clinician should consider how often these pauses have been occurring and how lengthy and complete the patient's narrative has been. If the patient has been limiting his remarks to a few phrases or sentences and then waiting for you to take the initiative again, you may have been interrogating him. If you have been asking a great many direct questions and continuing after brief replies, the patient will assume that brief replies in response to your questions are what you wish and expect. If, upon reflection, you feel you have placed yourself in such a situation, a pause on your part may encourage the patient to go on. If the patient continues to remain silent, it may be helpful to try a facilitating comment.

If, after reflecting on the course of the interview, you realize that you have been working hard to help the patient tell his story on his own, and you sense that the patient is "holding back" and that his nonverbal behavior reflects tension or discomfort, your silence is again likely to be appropriate. In the silence that follows, the patient's discomfort may well increase, and he may then tell you on his own what is bothering him and give you an opportunity to deal with it. This could be something in the immediate environment, such as telephone interruptions, the intrusion of office personnel, or a feeling that you are uninterested. On the other hand, it may be reticence, shame, or embarrassment about telling important parts of his story. The difficulty in communication that has developed may also be due to the patient's discomfort in speaking freely to someone of a different sex, age, class, race, or ethnic background. The patient may fear the possible diagnosis and react to this anxiety by failing to communicate freely in order to ward off the knowledge that he has the disease he dreads. Or his discomfort may be related to important events or circumstances in his personal life that you need to know about in order to manage his treatment successfully. Whatever the reason for the patient's evasiveness and discomfort, a pause will allow his discomfort to become clearly evident to both of you. If he does not speak about it spontaneously, you should be ready to point out the communication difficulities that you have been observing. A confrontation in this situation will frequently result in a discussion of the difficulty the patient is encountering. This will usually permit the interview to proceed smoothly.

When a patient has been communicating freely but then shows increasing difficulty with a particular topic and halts the account, his silence is best handled by remaining silent. In the ensuing pause, the emotional basis for the failure of communication may become apparent, and the clinician can then proceed with a confrontation leading to a discussion of the difficulty.

There is one time when it is mandatory for the clinician to remain silent. This is when the patient has stopped speaking because he or she is overwhelmed, or about to be overwhelmed, by emotion. When a patient begins to weep, especially if this progresses to sobbing, one must remain silent until he or she can regain some composure. Sometimes one may inhibit an expression of strong emotion—most frequently weeping—by prematurely saying something to the patient. There are several reasons for remaining silent until the patient has expressed the strong emotion and brought his feelings under control. Foremost is the fact that open expression of feelings almost always produces a relief of tension. In addition, it is likely that a patient will be able to express himself more adequately after a release of emotion. He may well be able to speak of things that he could not bring himself to discuss before. On the other hand, if the patient decides to control himself and withhold his feelings, he has the opportunity to do so. He makes the choice himself; it is not forced on him. The extent to which the patient is helped and the interview is facilitated by permitting a display of feeling depends very much on what the doctor says and does after it has subsided. A supportive response is almost always helpful. This will be taken up later in this chapter.

In some cases it will not be appropriate for you to remain silent when a patient pauses. If an overly talkative patient who had been dominating the interview and preventing the efficient gathering of diagnostic information stops talking, for example, you might take the opportunity to obtain some of the information you need. Another time when you would not necessarily remain silent at the patient's pause would be when you felt a need for clarification of what the patient had been saying. There are several ways you might choose to proceed. These will be described later.

In the early part of an interview, silence may allow the patient to go on to a new topic. If he shows signs of increasing tension as a silence develops, one can acknowledge what was just said, ask a broad question concerning this or other problems he may have, or comment on his discomfort. Near the close of the interview, when the interviewer feels he has a generally complete account of the patient's situation, he may not pause but instead immediately move on to obtain some specific information with questions.

There are a few "don'ts" with regard to the use of silence by the interviewer. Most individuals in our society are made uncomfortable by long silences in ordinary conversation. A doctor who overuses silence may be perceived by the patient as cold or distant. Certain individuals, particularly adolescents, do not tolerate silence well. When the interviewer perceives that his silence produces discomfort in the patient to the point of reducing further communication, he should become more active.

Confrontation

In confrontation the interviewer describes to the patient something striking about his or her verbal or nonverbal behavior. Here the clinician exerts a little more control over the direction the interview will take than he does in facilitation. Facilitation is a suggestion to the patient that he elaborate on a topic he has introduced, or simply go on with his story. Confrontation directs the patient's attention to something that he may be aware of only dimly or not at all. As a result, a confrontation very often has the effect of introducing a new topic. Examples of confrontations are: "You look sad," "You seem frightened," "You sound angry," "I notice that you have been rubbing the back of your neck." Like silence, confrontation may pose a difficult problem for the beginning student of interviewing. Students are often self-conscious about using it. In ordinary social conversation one does not call a person's attention to striking aspects of his manner or behavior that he is probably unaware of. To do so would usually be considered impolite. Very often, too, confrontation is a hostile act; it is commonly used in heated arguments. Since confrontation is not part of one's ordinary repertoire of social behaviors, one must practice its use as an effective expression of sympathy or support during an interview.

One situation in which a confrontation is useful occurs when the patient falls silent and is having difficulty continuing his or her account.

If there is a pause during which the patient's discomfort and perhaps its source have become evident, a confrontation is in order unless the patient ends the silence by describing his difficulties. The form of the confrontation will depend on what the interviewer has observed. Often useful are such comments as, "You seem to be having a good deal of difficulty telling me about this," or, "You appear quite uncomfortable." The patient who gives brief answers without elaborating may respond to the comment, "I notice you say very little except when I ask you questions." A common response is, "Oh, I didn't know you wanted me to go on." In other instances brief answers may be a sign of depression, and a confrontation may elicit information about that. At times, patients may be overcome with emotion and unable to voice their worries and fears. Confrontation can help them speak and afford them the relief of getting their concerns out in the open.

> The patient, a 55-year-old widowed woman, had a mastectomy for breast cancer four years earlier. As she described her symptoms of constant back pain, fatigue, and weight loss, she fell silent. Her facial expression and posture suggested worry and depression. She seemed close to tears.
>
> DOCTOR: (*softly, sympathetically*) You look like you're about to cry.
> (*Patient weeps softly, then dries her eyes.*)
> PATIENT: I promised myself I wouldn't do that but I couldn't help it. Every time I think it's the cancer coming back, I get so scared.

Note that in the above confrontation the interviewer describes how the patient appears to the interviewer. His comment is based on what he has observed. It does not make inferences about the patient's motives or her specific emotional state. Of course, it is possible that the interviewer has been incorrect in ascribing discomfort to the patient. In this case the remark will give the patient an opportunity to explain the difference between the clinician's perception of her behavior and her own. Such an explanation usually provides useful information.

The confrontation is not formulated as a question. At first glance, it might seem more efficient to ask, "Why are you uncomfortable?" or, "Why do you have so little to say?" There are several reasons for avoiding such questions. First, they are often felt by the patient to be a criticism. Second, they may not be an accurate perception. Third, a direct question also requires that the patient make some reply. The patient may not have developed sufficient trust in the doctor to reveal the required information or may not know or be able to formulate the answer to the question.

Another situation in which confrontation is useful occurs when the patient's nonverbal behavior communicates something to the interviewer that the patient is not talking about. For example, a housewife may be describing some set of physical symptoms while her doctor observes her dejected posture, the sad look about her eyes, her low and monotonous voice, and her twisting fingers. By some remark like, "It strikes me that you look very sad," the doctor responds to her nonverbal rather than her verbal communication. Slightly reddened eyes or trembling of the chin or lips may indicate that the patient is on the verge of tears. A sympathetic confrontation such as, "You look as if you are about to cry," may offer the patient an opportunity to give vent to his or her feelings of despair by open weeping. This may reduce the patient's tension and strengthen the relationship with the clinician. Physicians in particular tend to avoid situations that encourage a patient to cry for fear that the patient will later be ashamed or embarrassed about it. This fear very often stems from the doctor's own feelings about the shamefulness of crying. If the doctor responds to the weeping patient tactfully, it is very unlikely that the patient will feel ashamed or embarrassed. More likely, the patient will feel closer to the doctor.

Most clinicians, with the possible exception of psychiatrists, and almost all students are apprehensive about evoking too much emotional expression during a medical interview. Students will sometimes explain why they did not pick up on a very obvious nonverbal communication of emotion by saying, "I was afraid I would start the patient crying," or, "What do I do if the patient starts to cry?" The answer to the student's question is that one respectfully waits for the patient to finish crying and perhaps hands him a facial tissue, though not too quickly, as this might signal to the patient that he should not be crying. A supportive comment after an interval, such as, "I can see that you feel very bad about that," is also helpful. A similar acknowledgment of, say, anger ("I can see that you're very angry") is equally appropriate.

It is appropriate, too, to confront a patient when his voice, posture, body movement, or facial expression betray emotions such as anger or anxiety. One can say, "I get the impression that you are angry," or, "You sound angry." To an anxious patient one can say, "You look worried," or, "You seem tense," or one can remark on the behavior that betrays tension or anxiety by saying such things as, "I notice you're clenching your teeth," or, "You're trembling." All such remarks tend to promote a freer expression of feelings by the patient. Valuable information is derived and other needed information can be obtained more expeditiously after the patient expresses the despair, fear, anger, or other strong feeling. If the clinician handles the situation sensitively, the patient will feel increased trust and confidence.

The patient, a 62-year-old man, has a history of myocardial infarction at age 55.

DOCTOR: What kind of difficulties are you having?
PATIENT: I get these pains in my chest. (*He falls silent.*)
DOCTOR: Can you tell me more about them?
PATIENT: What else do you want to know? (*His hand goes to his face several times, touching his mouth. He remains silent.*)
DOCTOR: I notice you keep touching your face. You look very tense.
PATIENT: I am. I'm scared. I'm afraid of having another heart attack.

This patient was so fearful of another heart attack that he had difficulty talking about it, a not uncommon reaction. Calling attention to the behavioral signal of anxiety made it possible for him to talk about it. It was then relatively easy for him to describe his symptoms.

A supportive confrontation can also help to defuse anger, as in the following example:

A 39-year-old black woman on the diabetic service was sitting dangling her legs over the side of the bed as the student and the instructor approached the bed. The instructor introduced himself and the student to the patient and asked if she would agree to talk to the medical student about the troubles that brought her into the hospital. She agreed rather reluctantly.

The student, apparently not noticing that she had an amputation of the

right leg below the knee and loss of the great toe of the left foot, asked her
what sort of troubles she was having. She burst forth in a litany of angry,
profane remarks about the f—— hospital, the f—— doctors, and the
f—— nurses, etc.

While she was talking, the resident appeared at the foot of the bed and
told her she was going to surgery the next morning. He described the
procedure of removing the proximal part of the leg. She said angrily that
he could go to hell and that she was going to check herself out of the
hospital. He left.

The patient said she wanted to smoke, so the instructor wheeled her
outside. The student tried to start the interview again, but each question
was met with angry comments about her medical care, doctors in general,
and how she could take care of herself better on the outside. She said that it
was all the fault of her 13-year-old daughter, that she had come to the
hospital with a blister on her foot, was admitted, but two days later her
daughter was not obeying the patient's sister, who was looking after her
daughter, and that she had to leave in order to take care of her. The
student, looking helpless, felt she could go no further and turned to the
instructor. The instructor then commented that it sounded as if she had a
long history of being angry with doctors. The patient began to talk at once,
saying that she went into the hospital in diabetic coma at the age of nine
years, which was when her diabetes was discovered. The doctors, she said,
had lied to her, saying that by the age of 12 she wouldn't have to take
insulin anymore, and that this was the first of many lies. From age 12 to 36
she controlled her own diabetes. She had been seeing doctors ever since.
None of them ever had told the truth, she said. The more she talked, the
less angry she became. The interview ended when the nurse entered, told
her she now had to speak to the anesthesiologist, and wheeled her away.

The student, who was also black, admitted that she had been intimidated by the patient's anger and really didn't know what to do in the
interview. This is clearly a situation in which the obvious anger of this
anguished patient had to be dealt with at once. It is also an example of a
situation where an open-ended question is not the ideal way to open the
interview. Instead, the interviewer's attention should have been immediately drawn to the patient's expression of feeling as reflected in the
profanity with which she greeted the interviewer's open-ended question.

Observing the patient's behavior, including signs of tension, anxiety, depression, or anger, as revealed by expressions and movements, can be as important as obtaining the patient's story. When the patient's emotions stand out as prominently as they did in this example, the appropriate beginning is a supportively expressed confrontation such as, "You look very angry."

A particularly appropriate time to confront a patient is when his verbal and nonverbal behavior are clearly incongruent. For example, a patient may speak about very sad things in an indifferent manner, about insults of gross injustice without displaying anger, or about comfortable circumstances and happy events in a mood of dejection. A comment on these discrepancies may lead to valuable information about the patient's difficulties and conflicts. A confrontation is also appropriate when there are inconsistencies in the patient's story. This almost always leads to valuable information.

> In describing the problem that caused him to seek medical help, the 62-year-old patient said he had had episodes of chest pain radiating into his left arm provoked by heavy exertion. As the interview continued, he mentioned, almost in passing, that once when he got up from his desk to walk across his office he had the same symptoms.
>
> DOCTOR: I'm a little puzzled about that. A little while ago you said this happens with heavy exertion. But walking a few steps doesn't sound like heavy exertion. Can you help me to understand that?
>
> PATIENT: Well, now that I think about it, it happens more often now and it doesn't take as much exertion to bring it on. As a matter of fact, yesterday I went up two steps into the entrance of my building and I got the pain.

There are a few cautions to be stated about confrontations. In ordinary conversation, when we speak of confronting someone we often mean a hostile accusation. The term often has an unpleasant connotation of anger, even though there are many types of positive confrontations. When confrontations are made in an interview, they should reflect sympathetic interest in the patient. Sometimes the interviewer's irriation with the patient's behavior may be the cue that calls this behavior to his attention, but it is his interest in this peculiarity of behavior and in furthering the goals of the interview that should prompt and be expressed in the confrontation.

A second caution concerns the overuse of confrontation. Even though the patient is confronted in a sympathetic manner, he may feel criticized if he is confronted too often. Confrontations can develop a nagging quality. No more than one or two confrontations based on the same or related observations are appropriate in any interview.

Sometimes at the outset of an interview a patient is in obvious distress and is signaling it by body language such as rubbing an affected joint with a look of pain or giving signs of respiratory distress. In this case it is appropriate to begin the interview with a confrontation. While technically a confrontation, it is actually an acknowledgment of the patient's distress and indicates concern for the patient. This will be discussed in greater detail later in this chapter.

Questions

The closed-ended question, which specifies the area of information desired, is controlling and limiting. Open-ended questions, on the other hand, are much less controlling and are usually facilitating.

Questions that require a very specific answer are rarely appropriate if the interviewer does not know how he will use the information in arriving at a decision. If direct questions are properly phrased, answers will most often be brief but high in information content.

Beginning students of interviewing often ask questions out of discomfort when a patient falls silent. Such questions are more likely to interfere with communication than to encourage it. With increasing self-confidence and a sense of purpose in undertaking the interview, students soon find it less necessary to ask many closed-ended questions.

There is an important role for asking questions in an interview and an appropriate time and style for questions. These will be discussed in detail in Chapter 3.

The most controlling questions are those that call for a yes or no answer. A similar form is the multiple-choice query in which the interviewer specifies a list of specific replies he expects the patient to choose from: "Does this pain come on before, after, or during meals?" These two types of questions may be called *checklist questions*, since they are a verbal equivalent of the kind of questions that may be answered by checking off a preprinted response on a questionnaire.

Checklist questions are generally to be avoided in the open-ended part of the interview. Both types tend to stop the interchange. The patient "checks off" his reply and waits for the next question. Furthermore, both types tend to suggest that the interviewer is not interested in information that does not fall into the categories provided and expects the patient to "pigeonhole" his reply categorically. More communicative patients may overcome this suggestion and provide relevant information not requested, but the interviewer should not rely on this when formulating questions. It is particularly difficult to create good multiple-choice questions spontaneously. The categories should be exhaustive and mutually exclusive. If all possible alternatives are not offered, bias is introduced. If all alternatives are presented, the question is likely to be so complex that it will confuse the patient. Multiple-choice questions, therefore, are best given in written form. Questioning is the interviewing behavior most likely to produce biased information. A discussion of ways to avoid bias will be found in Chapter 3.

At what points in the interview is it wise to use direct questions? The first is anytime one cannot get needed information with a lower degree of control. The second is when the broad outlines of the story have emerged and specific information about details is needed. These include the review of systems, inquiry into past illnesses, and parts of the mental status examination. Chapter 3 will deal with these aspects of the interview.

Direction

This is the highest use of control. Directions are statements that instruct the patient what he should say or do. Sometimes directions can be facilitating. Directions to speak, such as, "Tell me more about that," are not very controlling because they do not limit the range of information that the patient is asked to give to anything like the degree that a direct and highly specific question does. Thus, directions, too, can allow a patient considerable latitude in what he says. Of course, directions are a necessary part of the physical examination.

Suggestion

Somewhat less control than with either questions or directions is exercised when the interviewer makes a *suggestion*. A suggestion is a subtle direction that may guide the patient's thinking or behavior. Because of the authority of the clinician, it will have much more effect on the patient than the same words would have in a different setting. For this reason, suggestion is the most common way of biasing information. This can be done in several ways. One is by the wording of the question. Another is by shifting topics, which may say to the patient, "That's not important—no more about that." It can also be done by interpreting what the patient has said, or by mentioning a tentative diagnosis. Suggesting a pattern of pain or a symptom must be avoided in diagnostic interviewing. However, suggestion may be helpful in treatment; it is probably the basis of the placebo effect.

How is suggestion best used by the interviewer? The answer is that it should be part of a facilitating comment. For example, when the clinician picks up on something the patient has just said by repeating it, he is suggesting that the patient pursue that topic further.

Suggestion can be harmful to patients when done improperly. Such comments as, "This is a very serious problem," or any statement that sounds ominous such as, "You mean you waited this long before coming in?" can frighten the patient, creating unnecessary anxiety.

Support and Reassurance

Trust and confidence in the clinician are built when the patient is offered support. Support refers to behavior on the part of the interviewer that reflects an attitude of interest, concern, and positive regard or respect for the patient. Supportive statements, such as, "I understand," or, "That must have been very upsetting," convey sympathetic comprehension of what the patient has just said. Particularly after expressions of strong feelings such as anger, fear, or worry, support is appreciated by the patient. It enhances the solidarity of the relationship and helps the patient to continue his account.

Supportive words must be spontaneous and genuine to be helpful. If overdone or too studied and unspontaneous, they will fail to accomplish their intended purpose because the patient will perceive them as insincere.

Reassurance may be supportive if used appropriately. Reassurance refers to words or acts designed to restore the patient's confidence or diminish the patient's fears. Here, too, the clinician's attitude must convey reassurance, not just his words. To be effective, reassurance must be based on evidence or fact and must be genuine. Clichés are rarely reassuring.

But reassurance should not be given in a way that creates unreasonable expectations. To promise that everything will turn out well is a poor use of reassurance unless the evidence clearly supports such a statement. The statement, "You are making satisfactory progress," is reassuring only if it is based on good evidence that the patient can understand.

NONVERBAL COMMUNICATION

Communication goes on between clinician and patient whether or not one or the other is speaking, as in all face-to-face interactions. Thus far, this chapter has dealt primarily with verbal communication. Nonverbal communication, or body language, can be even more important than the words that are spoken.

The nonverbal communication that takes place between two or more people was called "the silent language" by Hall.[4] Information about the patient's emotional status can be obtained from both verbal and nonverbal behavior, and at times nonverbal behavior is essential to understanding what the patient is trying to say. Understanding nonverbal behavior requires that the interviewer carefully observe the patient's gait, demeanor, posture, facial expression, tone of voice, etc. throughout the interview and during the physical examination. Taking notes and looking at one's chart or clipboard while writing is a common barrier to "reading" body language. Even more frequent, however, is the simple failure to observe the patient carefully and to heed the communication that is not being provided in words. This may happen because many clinicians are less comfortable with patients' feelings than they are with "facts," such as descriptions of symptoms and their time of onset. Anger, sadness, resentment, and fear are also facts, though some clinicians prefer not to deal with them. They may be as relevant to an understanding of the clinical problem as more "objective" data.

A useful exercise to increase observational skill and descriptive accuracy is to diagram the interview, separating observations of behavior and expressions of feelings from the elements of the patient's account. In this exercise the data may be listed in two columns. All the nonverbal signs are placed in one column. Everything the patient talked about is put into the second column in a series of summarizing statements. This would include the topics the patient brought up, the story of the illness, and information given about needs, preoccupations, and goals. An example of such an analysis follows:

Mr. H. was a 55-year-old manufacturer's representative who had been employed for many years by a large corporation until he was laid off approximately six months before this examination. His layoff had been part of a personnel cutback caused by economic conditions. He had had abdominal discomfort and ulcer-like pain for a few years that he had managed to control by using over-the-counter antacids. After his layoff, his alcohol intake increased and he began to have more abdominal discomfort. He described his symptoms during the interview and mentioned the fact that he had been quite tense for several years before losing his job. Since that time he had become depressed, uncertain, indecisive, and obsessively preoccupied with his feelings of betrayal by his former employer and with his physical symptoms.

The interviewer noted to himself that the patient looked to be at least ten years older than his 55 years. His facial expression was one of uncertainty and sadness. He had a downturned mouth and looked down at the floor. He spoke softly and expressed pessimism about his ability to find work at his age and in an economic recession. His shoulders drooped. He volunteered little and answered questions only after pauses and in a soft voice.

The material in this example has been listed in Table 2.2. The advantage of organizing the behavioral data in this way is obvious. By reviewing the ten points listed in the observations column, one can see at once that this patient is very depressed. It is also obvious that the diagnosis of depression is as necessary to his treatment as the diagnosis that will come from careful investigation of his abdominal symptoms.

TABLE 2.2. Analysis of an Interview

Observations	Content
1. Sad facial expression	1. 55-year-old businessman
2. Downturned mouth	2. Upper abdominal sharp
3. Looks down	pains relieved by antacids
4. Drooping shoulders	3. Lost job
5. Soft voice	4. Expresses feelings of
6. Volunteers little	betrayal
7. Moves and speaks slowly	5. Loss of interest in life
8. Demeanor communicates	6. Feels indecisive
pessimism	7. Worried about the future
9. Acts indecisively	
10. Initiates no actions	
and waits for examiner	
to ask a question	

Facial Expressions

Sadness is often mirrored in the face of the depressed patient. A down-turned mouth, lackluster eyes, or a slight quivering at the point of the chin or lower lip are signs of sadness. Clenched teeth with bulging masseters indicate tension, sometimes due to anger. A fixed smile implies that the patient is anxious to please you and may be fearful. Sometimes a forced smile is used to mask depression and to fight off a desire to weep. Such a smile does not include the eyes and seems hollow. Simply pointing out the unconvincing smile may help the patient clarify the underlying meaning. One can say, "You're smiling but you don't look very happy!" Anxiety usually shows in a patient's face as a discernible look of apprehension, often accompanied by rapid, shallow breathing. The apprehensive patient often has darting eye movements and looks about the room and without maintaining eye contact except for brief periods. Physical pain can be communicated through facial expressions, even when the patient is not fully conscious.

A person's eyes can be quite revealing. Depression shows there. Eye contact that is too intense may occur when the patient glares at the in-

terviewer (anger) or attempts to be seductive (manipulative behavior)—
expressions which, of course, are not difficult to tell apart. Inability to
maintain eye contact may reflect guilt feelings, as when a guilt-laden
topic is being discussed. It may also indicate anxiety or the patient's
difficulty in coping with his feelings about the interviewer. Normally,
when patients are listening carefully or are intent on telling their story,
they will look directly at the interviewer but will not appear apprehensive
or angry unless those feelings are being immediately experienced in
response to what is being discussed. They will not, however, give an
impression of staring at the interviewer.

Posture

The patient's posture communicates something of his attitude toward
you, and of his dominant emotion. Posture can reflect openness (relaxed arms at sides, slightly slouched in the chair) or a closed, defensive, distrustful attitude (arms closed, hugging oneself, sitting up very
straight). Slumped shoulders and a bowed head are marks of depression.
Anxiety is often signaled by the patient's shifting about, tapping fingers,
moving feet and legs, or gripping the arms of a chair with white
knuckles.

Note whether the patient leans away from you or shifts his chair to
increase the distance (thereby indicating defensiveness or distrust) or
leans toward you or moves closer (implying a desire for more intimacy).
There are also ethnic differences in the distance from others that one
finds comfortable. For example, people from Latin cultures may move
closer to you than those of Anglo-Saxon heritage.

If a patient's posture reveals belligerence, this attitude must be dealt
with, as it can be a deterrent to a successful interview. It is best to call
attention to it in a tactful, nonthreatening way so that it can be brought
out into the open and discussed.

A 43-year-old construction worker was being seen for evaluation in the
Rehabilitation Medicine clinic. The interviewer noticed that the patient's
fists were clenched, his jaws tightly clenched, and that he sat stiffly erect.
He said, "I can't help but notice how you are sitting. You look like you

don't want to be here." "I don't," said the patient, and went on to describe, with considerable anger, the great number of examinations he had had and his feeling that he was considered to be either a hypochondriac or a malingerer. After the interviewer reassured him that he held no such attitude and that the ultimate purpose of the interview was to initiate treatment, the patient relaxed and the interview proceeded uneventfully.

Tone of Voice

We all know that the same words spoken in two different tones of voice may have very different meanings. If asked how one's day has been, a reply of, "Just fine," said in a warm and pleasant tone usually means just that; the same words said quickly, tonelessly, and without conviction may really mean, "Don't bother me. I've had a bad day and I don't want to talk about it." When interviewing a patient, especially on follow-up visits or after an interval of some length since the previous interview, the response to the usual inquiry about how the patient has been feeling may be just such a brief comment. The intonation of the words may then be the clue to how the patient feels. It may also indicate the patient's attitude toward the interviewer or the need for further encounters with health care providers. The interviewer's response is usually keyed more to the nonverbal communication of the patient's tone of voice than to the content of the words. Alertness to the intonation and a simple comment or query about it may open up a whole vein of useful information.

Gestures

Valuable information about patients' feelings can be obtained by observing their gestures. These are often involuntary and probably instinctive, though how pronounced and expressive they are is influenced by the culture from which the patient comes. Covering the eyes or mouth may mean, "I don't want to see it," or, "I don't want to talk." Reaching out to put a hand on the interviewer's arm or to finger his coat lapel may mean, "Listen to me," or, "Pay more attention to me." Shrugs, waggling the palm of the hand, or holding the palm outward toward the interviewer are easily read messages that usually emphasize the speaker's words or can substitute for a verbal message. When a patient rubs or repeatedly touches a part of his body, one should comment on or inquire about it. The motion usually means pain or discomfort in that area. Anxiety is often signaled by gestures such as rubbing the chin, pulling at the lip, twisting fingers, or tapping fingers or feet. A typical gesture of the frightened, guilt-ridden, or worried person is the partial elevation of one shoulder or the arm as though preparing to ward off a blow.

A study of nonverbal expressions of anxiety during patient interviews by family practitioners demonstrated that what the authors termed "hand-to-body self-touching" occurred significantly more often while patients were talking about anxiety-producing topics.[5] Other gestures that illustrated what the patients were talking about did not differ in frequency whether the patients were speaking about anxiety-provoking matters or more neutral ones. In short, if the patient frequently touches some part of his body with his hand, he is probably feeling anxiety.[6] Such behavior should be noted. An appropriate comment after a sufficient number of observations might be, "You look very tense," or, "You look very anxious."

Congruence

Any nonverbal message from the patient that suggests something other than the content of the verbal message or seems to be in conflict with it should be given special attention. As we have said, gestures, facial expressions, posture, and tone of voice are more reliable indicators of feelings and attitudes than words. Since verbal messages are under conscious control, they are subject to censorship and may be used for purposes of persuasion, to mislead others, or to hide what one does not wish to reveal. But body language is not so easily censored and will usually give reliable indications of the patient's emotional state. Lack of congruence between verbal and nonverbal messages may indicate that something significant is being omitted, whether deliberately or unconsciously. Thus, the skilled interviewer who notes a discrepancy between the verbal and nonverbal messages will inquire about it. An effective way of doing this is through confrontation. For example, "You know,

Mr. Smith, you say you feel just fine but you look very unhappy." This will frequently focus the patient's attention on his mood. Much new information may then emerge. When patients have difficulty facing certain problems and are attempting to keep their concerns out of their consciousness, their words may serve to help them do that. Their involuntary body expressions will help you decipher the hidden message and bring the patients to an awareness of problems for which there may be some treatment.

CONCLUSION

The open-ended interview, in summary, represents a style of interviewing that is most likely to create a patient-centered rather than a physician-centered interview. The traditional medical interview emphasizes data collection and aims for high efficiency in gathering detailed data within limited time periods. The open-ended interview emphasizes attention to rapport and to the development of the clinician-patient relationship. It aims to facilitate the emergence of facts rather than their extraction from the patient, thereby creating the opportunity for less biased and more relevant information, both verbal and nonverbal. It relies on a differential use of the clinician's authority, never using more authority than is required to get the needed data, and on the ability of the interviewer, through appropriate support and reassurance, to express his or her interest in helping the patient.

REFERENCES

1. Gill, M., R. Newman, and F. C. Redlich, *The Initial Interview in Psychiatric Practice*. New York: International Universities Press, 1954.
2. Enelow, A. J., L. M. Adler, and P. Manning, "A Supervised Psychotherapy Course for Practicing Physicians," *Journal of Medical Education*, 39:140–146, 1964.
3. Payne, S. L., *The Art of Asking Questions*. Princeton, N.J.: Princeton University Press, 1951.

4. Hall, Edward T., *The Silent Language*. Garden City, N.Y.: Doubleday, 1959.

5. Shreve, E. G., J. A. Harrigan, J. R. Kues, and D. N. Kagas, "Non-verbal Expressions of Anxiety in Physician-Patient Interactions," *Psychiatry*, 51:378–384, 1988.

6. Harrigan, J. A., "Self-touching as an Indicator of Underlying Affect and Language Process," *Social Science and Medicine*, 20:1161–1168, 1985.

3

THE MEDICAL HISTORY

KEY POINTS

1. Chief complaints are often a mixture of the stated reason to see the doctor and underlying psychological or social concerns.
2. The chronological presentation of the history may meander, but the interviewer can guide it.
3. Open-ended interviewing techniques should be used early in the interview, followed by direct inquiry.
4. The past history elicits conditions that may have caused present or future illness.
5. Sexual history and substance abuse are topics that must be elicited by the interviewer, rather than waiting for the patient to bring them up.

The medical history provides 70 to 80 percent of the information for most diagnoses. It has several components: the chief complaint, the history of the present illness, the past medical history, the family history, and the review of symptoms. Together with the sexual history and, where relevant, the history of drug or alcohol abuse, these provide a story of a patient's life that is essential to an understanding of his health and the illness for which he is being seen by the physician. An open-ended interview, as described in Chapter 2, will uncover that story.

As the patient talks about his pain and the suffering and losses it has caused him, the clinician, using facilitation, confrontation, support, and questions, will clarify this story. As noted in Chapter 1, experienced clinicians may strongly suspect the cause of the patient's problems from this information alone. But a patient's story is always larger than the present problem. The past illness history, family background, work history, and daily activities will all play a role in deciding how to treat the patient.

This chapter addresses the major components of the medical history (Table 3.1). What is a "chief" complaint? How does the clinician uncover the intricacies of the present illness? How should one find out about the patient's past life? The answers to these questions are found through skillful open-ended interviewing, supplemented by direct questions when needed.

CHIEF COMPLAINTS

The symptoms responsible for the patient seeking medical help are called the *chief complaint*. Patients may have one chief complaint or more. In the following examples, the patients expressed a single chief complaint:

A 73-year-old retired physicist wondered why he had an unexplained six-pound weight loss during the previous month.

A 46-year-old businessman reported severe pain in the right great toe that had awakened him six hours earlier.

TABLE 3.1. Components of a Complete History

1. Chief complaints
2. Present illness
3. Past medical history
4. Sexual history
5. Substance use and abuse
6. Family history
7. Review of systems

A 40-year-old nurse, who worked in a doctor's office, complained of the sudden onset of a "migraine" headache.

But there are almost always other significant problems, as seen in the next example:

A 29-year-old single, African-American classical ballet dancer who was interviewed in a county hospital complained of sore, swollen joints. She had been well until three months earlier when she was unable to get out of bed because of pain in her ankles and knees. Her fingers and wrists were swollen and she couldn't raise her arms above her head because of pain. The doctor, who had treated her various dance injuries, told her to take Advil, and to "stay in touch." She did not improve and did not see a physician because she had lost her medical insurance when she was terminated by the ballet company. Her boyfriend, with whom she had lived for two years, told her she complained too much. After three months of illness, she flew home to her mother because, "I always go home to my mother when I get depressed." He mother took her to an Emergency Room, and, lacking insurance, the patient was admitted to the county hospital.

Patients usually have several chief complaints. The dancer not only complained of pain and swelling of several joints, but was tired, irritable, and frightened. She had become depressed and came home to her mother for the emotional support she was not receiving from her boyfriend. Complaints are often of a physical nature though there are usually psychosocial or economic factors that help prompt the patient to seek medical attention. The retired physicist with sudden weight loss feared he might have cancer. The businessman with the painful toe was scheduled to leave on a business trip. The nurse couldn't work because of her migraine.

When a patient has several complaints, it can be difficult to decide which are the primary ones. Asking the question, "What finally led to your coming for help?" will often elicit the chief reason for the office or clinic visit. Frequently, the most important complaint is the first symptom mentioned by the patient, such as, "I can't walk because of the pain in my hip and I'm afraid it might be arthritis."

Balint[1] suggested that patients need a medical complaint in order to warrant medical attention, that having a medical symptom legitimizes the clinical encounter. Patients often present with a sore throat, a simple cold, or some other complaint. The clinician may wonder why the patient has bothered to seek help for minor symptoms. The disparity between the patient's concern and the mildness of the complaint should alert the clinician to the possibility of an underlying reason for the medical visit. Barsky[2] referred to such underlying concerns, which only emerge after the patient has talked about other less serious problems, as the "hidden reasons" patients visit the doctor.

A common hidden reason patients see doctors is depression. They may casually refer to being depressed in the course of describing a minor illness. Or they may wait until the clinician comments on how sad they seem before revealing the real reason for coming to the doctor.

A 35-year-old married, Caucasian housewife voiced the chief complaint of difficulty in getting through the day because of fatigue. Several months earlier she had begun to notice that she felt tired when she awakened in the morning. The fatigue had increased to the point of exhaustion. Concerned that she might have low thyroid function or be anemic, she made an appointment to see her doctor.

This patient had been denying her depression since she first felt fatigue several months earlier. She really thought she was just very, very tired. When the physician said, "Mrs. Jones, you look so very sad when you tell me about your fatigue," she broke down in tears and told the story of her husband's infidelity and her depression.

Fear is another hidden reason for seeing a doctor, as in the following example:

A 28-year-old single man visited the doctor because of a month's history of "spasms" in his penis when he started to urinate. There were no accompanying symptoms to suggest either a urinary tract infection or a sexually transmitted disease. As he became more comfortable in telling his story, he revealed that he had had unprotected sex with a prostitute four months earlier at a time when he was having ambivalent feelings about his girlfriend, with whom he had a four-year monogamous relationship. He was filled with fear that he might have contracted a sexually transmitted disease, which he might give to his girlfriend, and with guilt about his infidelity. He was trying to wait six months before having an AIDS test, but his concern about the urinary symptom drove him to seek medical help.

The chief complaints may reveal the reason that the patient is sick or the organ system involved. For example, a patient with shaking chills, high fever, cough productive of bloody sputum, and pleuritic chest pain has a pulmonary problem, most likely pneumonia. The chief complaints alone will often enable the clinician to make a presumptive diagnosis. Burack[3] found that the presenting complaint predicted the principal medical problem 60 percent of the time. Nevertheless, up to 40 percent of the time the presenting chief complaints focused attention on issues that did not turn out to be the major problem.

Not all patients seek the physician's attention for relief of medical complaints. The reason for the visit may be a pre-employment or annual physical examination, and the patient may be in excellent health, entirely free of symptoms. Some patients may be seen for routine blood pressure monitoring or a cholesterol check. Middle-aged men and women often want or are required to have a treadmill examination before starting an exercise program. Even in these situations, however, it is important to be alert to possible hidden anxieties. For instance, the 40-year-old man scheduled for a treadmill test may be worried about his heart because of a strong family history of heart disease.

In discussing a patient's illness with a colleague or in recording the medical history, the interviewer begins with an identifying statement and description of the chief complaints. This includes the patient's age, sex, race, marital status, and the reason for seeking medical attention. For example:

The patient is a 32-year-old, single, Caucasian male security guard who has been using alcohol and cocaine to excess in the past year and in the past three months has complained of constant thirst, urinating night and day, and a slight loss of weight despite being hungry and eating a lot.

The identifying statement tells us something about the patient with the illness. The chief complaints tell us why he has sought medical attention. Together, they give a quick overview of the patient and his medical problems.

PRESENT ILLNESS

The *present illness* is the account of the problems for which a person seeks medical help (Table 3.2). Of the various components of a medical history, it is the most important. It usually has both medical and psychosocial features. The process of eliciting those features is begun by establishing the time of onset of the present illness.

Onset of the Present Illness

The onset of the present illness may be sudden or gradual. Most common infectious diseases have a sudden beginning. The patient may be able to recall the exact day or hour when symptoms such as chills, fever, and sweats began. On the other hand, when the illness has a slow, insidious onset, it may be difficult for patients to remember when the symptoms first appeared. This is particularly true of so-called constitutional symptoms. These are complaints such as loss of appetite and weight, or easy fatigability, that are not characteristic of one particular disease but are common to many. These symptoms of insidious onset are often seen in patients with cancer, endocrine disorders, and chronic infections. The patient with a cancer may initially notice a weight loss, the patient with thyroid disease may complain of unusual tiredness, and

TABLE 3.2. Components of the Present Illness

1. Onset of the present illness
2. Chronology
3. "WH" questions
4. Closure
5. Transition to past history

the patient with a chronic infection of low-grade fever, fatigue, and sweats. Patients with AIDS may complain of swollen lymph glands, unusual skin lesions, fever, or a host of other nonspecific symptoms. In many of these disorders, it may be difficult to date the onset of the present illness. The following is such an example:

> The patient, a 51-year-old insurance broker, had a long history of heart disease culminating in coronary artery bypass surgery in 1981. He remained well until 1993 when he had a cardiac arrest, was resuscitated, and had a defibrillator implanted in his abdomen. About that same time, he had a prostatic abscess which, though very resistant to antibiotic treatment, finally responded. During all of this time, the physician's attention was almost completely focused on his cardiac problems. After these were controlled and the prostatic abscess was cured, the patient began to experience chills and high fever. Efforts to identify the cause of these symptoms were not successful. Then his wife, an R.N., recalled that he had been having unexplained sweats and fevers for several years. This additional information prompted the physician to order an HIV test, which was positive. The patient had contracted the virus 10 years earlier from a blood transfusion at the time of the open heart surgery. Before the cause of the opportunistic infection could be discovered, he died of a cardiac arrest. The autopsy indicated he had disseminated tuberculosis.

This example illustrates the difficulties the clinician may encounter in trying to date the onset of a new illness. If it is not quite clear when the illness began, the interviewer may ask the patient when he was last in good health. The patient might then remember that he was in good health at the time of a birthday, anniversary, or during a significant holiday as in the following story.

> A 68-year-old, widowed psychologist complained of being exhausted but had difficulty in pinpointing the onset of this symptom. She recalled feeling well during the Christmas holidays two months earlier. She remembered telling her son, who is a physician, of pain in her hip for which he prescribed a nonsteroidal anti-inflammatory drug. While the medication relieved her hip pain, she discontinued it after ten days because of burning pain in her upper abdomen. She then remembered that this was

about the time she became so exhausted. She appeared pale to the interviewer and was found to be severely anemic due to blood loss from a bleeding gastric ulcer caused by the drug she had taken for her hip pain.

While it is important to know when the present illness began, at the beginning of the interview it is best to encourage the patient to relate his story without interruption. Becoming too concerned about the timing of events early in the interview may reduce that patient's spontaneity and prepare him for a question-and-answer format. The interviewer can always return later to the task of identifying the exact time of onset of the illness.

In response to the kind of open-ended inquiry described in Chapter 2, a patient will usually give a very brief description of his illness. The studies of Beckman and Frankel[4] show that if a patient is uninterrupted, he will seldom continue on his own for more than a couple of minutes. Then most patients will pause. The inexperienced interviewer may think the patient has finished his spontaneous account and begin to ask specific questions. More likely, the patient is looking to the interviewer to help him tell his story. By a simple nod of the head or the use of one of several facilitating responses such as, "I see," or "Go on," known linguistically as continuers, the physician can usually encourage the patient to continue his story. If for some reason the patient does not continue, the interviewer can briefly recap what he has heard. The patient will then be likely to add additional details or offer new material. Sometimes when the patient's beginning story has been emotionally laden, a supportive comment such as, "I can see you have been through a lot," will encourage the patient to continue on his own.

Often the patient's appearance will indicate physical or emotional distress. In such instances, the interviewer should consider opening the interview with an empathic comment (supportive confrontation) indicating his awareness of the patient's distress. To begin the interview with an open-ended question might be inappropriate. One would not ask the patient who is wheezing and struggling for breath what sort of troubles he is having. Rather, the interviewer would remark on the patient's obvious difficulty. Similarly, patients who appear sad or anxious may welcome acknowledgment of their distress rather than being asked what brought them into the hospital or clinic.

In the hospital setting, patients are frequently getting in or out of bed, eating their meals, having blood drawn, or conversing with family members or friends when the interviewer arrives on the scene. Or the patient may be asleep and is awakened for the interview. These situations provide the opportunity to begin the interview on a human level by acknowledging the circumstances at the time of the interview. Such a statement reflecting consideration of the patient's feelings allows the interview to start more naturally. The clinician can usually be forgiven for awakening a patient if he apologizes for his action. Commenting on the patient's discomfort or pain after blood has been withdrawn is a more sensitive beginning than asking the patient what sort of troubles he has been having.

Patients who appear anxious as they begin to tell the story of their illness may have difficulty at first with open-ended questions. Providing a little more structure initially will often relieve some of their anxiety. Acknowledging their anxiety or asking them to tell something about themselves can help to make them more comfortable. After a few structured questions, one can use a more open-ended style.

Chronology of the Present Illness

Early in the interview the patient is likely to describe his or her symptoms in a helter-skelter fashion without regard to chronology. The task of the interviewer is to create order out of disorder. This is done by carefully reviewing what the patient has said. Such mini-summaries shape the story so that it can be followed from its beginning to its end. This is illustrated in the following example.

The patient was a 38-year-old Caucasian married computer operator who was holding her abdomen and was clearly in great pain when the clinician came to her bedside. He began the interview by saying that he could see she was in a lot of pain. The patient responded by telling him that she hurt, was sick at her stomach, had been vomiting, and thought it was all because she couldn't move her bowels. He determined that she had first become sick about 36 hours earlier. She referred to abdominal pain, pointing to her upper abdomen. As she continued to speak of her nausea, cramps and feelings of concern, the doctor began to sort out the story as follows:

DOCTOR: Now as I understand it, Mrs. Brown, this all started with pain just above the navel.

PATIENT: Well, I woke up about three o'clock in the morning with pain right here (*points again to the mid-upper abdomen*). I couldn't sleep. Then I got sick to my stomach and vomited.

DOCTOR: You got sick to your stomach and vomited.

PATIENT: Yes. The pain was awful. It kept getting worse. I tried to get up and go to work but I couldn't. I thought maybe it was my bowels, but when I tried to go to the bathroom I couldn't have a bowel movement.

DOCTOR: And then?

PATIENT: It went on all day and that night, too. By this morning the pain was down on my right side. (*The patient fell silent.*)

DOCTOR: It all started, then, with pain just above the navel the night before last about three o'clock in the morning. Then you began to vomit. You tried to move your bowels but nothing happened, and then the pain moved down into your lower right side.

PATIENT: Yes. I just want something for the pain. It was so bad, I could hardly move. I felt hot. I took my temperature and it was over 100 degrees. And it still hurts, doctor.

The patient was helped to tell her story by short summaries and facilitating remarks such as, "And then?"

Most illnesses have a characteristic chronology as they progress from their onset to the point when the patient consults a physician. Occasionally patients may be seen early in the course of an illness before an identifiable chronology has developed. For example, Herpes zoster characteristically presents as pain in the area of one or more dermatomes of the body and persists for days before the skin eruption appears. The diagnosis is suggested by the distribution of pain, but only the appearance of the blisters will confirm this suspicion.

Some patients, such as children and teenagers, have more difficulty than others in providing a chronological description of illness. They are likely to use one or two words to describe how they feel. Direct questioning will help put the story together. They may complain of pain, for example, without concern for the time of its beginning or its course. On the other hand, a garrulous patient may talk at great length about both his medical and psychosocial problems without paying much attention to their relevance to his current problem. The interviewer will have to become more directive to help the patient back on track. A statement like, "The story of your sister's wedding is interesting, but I'd like to know more about your weight loss," will help the patient focus on current problems. Older patients with cognitive disorders may have difficulty providing a sequential history due to impaired short-term memory. Those with psychotic thought disorders may have such loose associations between one thought and the next that following the story becomes very difficult for the interviewer. In these instances one may have to depend heavily on family members or others to provide the needed information.

While listening intently to the story of medical illness and attempting to understand its chronology, it is important not to miss the personal story. Clues to psychosocial problems may be found in chance remarks such as, "Things have not been going well lately," or, "I've been having these headaches ever since my wife died." The way the patient refers to a spouse, family member, of friend may suggest a troubled relationship. By reflecting such remarks back to the patient, either when first heard or later in the interview, the clinician is telling the patient that he is just as concerned about these issues as about the medical ones. These non-medical clues have been referred to as "windows of opportunity."[5] In almost every interview, even one of short duration with a biomedical focus, the interviewer can utilize windows of opportunity to explore psychosocial issues.

Beginning the interview in an open-ended way will allow the clinician to see the broad perspective of the present illness. But a point will be reached when the clinician must ask specific questions to obtain more information about a problem that has been tentatively identified. This is the moment when the interview changes from being patient-centered to physician-centered.[6]

Direct Inquiry and Avoiding Bias

Direct inquiry should be conducted in a manner that does not bias the resulting communication. Accuracy in communication is facilitated when the interviewer does not suggest responses to the patient by his wording of questions, tone of voice, or other nonverbal communication. The interviewer's manner can be a source of bias. Facial expressions or gestures that convey moral judgements, surprise, or a greatly accentuated interest or attention will influence what the patient tells or does not tell. The wording of the interviewer's communication can also reveal his own biases and thereby influence the patient's account.

It is best to begin direct inquiry with general questions and gradually move to more specific, detailed questions, a process called *narrowing*.[7] It is better to ask, "When does the pain come on?" before asking, "Does the pain come on right after meals?" As the interviewer seeks more detailed information, it becomes increasingly difficult to formulate open-ended questions. Therefore, as questions become highly specific, alternatives should be offered to the patient. Behavioral science research on question wording[8] has shown that questions like, "Does the pain come on right after meals?" will elicit more "Yes" responses than will a question like, "Does the pain come on right after meals, or do you notice it at other times?" In wording a question, one should give each alternative equal weight as in, "Does exertion bring on the pain, or do you notice it at times when you have not been exerting yourself?"

It is most important to formulate questions in a way that does not suggest an expected answer or pattern of pain. Thus, "Does the pain stay in one place or does it travel?" is better than, "Does the pain shoot down your leg?" Confrontation may be used to avoid the introduction of bias. For example, if the patient repeatedly rubs some part of the body, such as the knee, it is better to use confrontation, such as, "I notice that you're rubbing your knee," than to ask, "Does your knee hurt?"

The timing of questions and of shifts in topics can also introduce bias. It is important to avoid interpretations or suggestions about the nature of the problem during the information-gathering phases of the interview. One should not pursue a specific line of inquiry longer than really necessary or to the exclusion of other unexplored areas. Excessive and highly detailed concentration on one area or line of inquiry will often convince the patient that there must be something wrong there.

Questioning should always be framed for the specific patient being interviewed, taking into account his language skills, social and cultural background, and style of communication. With all patients one should use simple, concise, nontechnical language that the patient understands.

Developing a Line of Inquiry

When the clinician decides to seek specific information, it is best obtained by gradually restricting the open-endedness of the series of questions presented to the patient. In the following example, the patient has mentioned "tiredness" as his main problem:

DOCTOR: You say you're really tired?

PATIENT: Well, I was okay until about two weeks ago when I could hardly get throught the day I was so tired. This is about the same time I noticed all the bruises on my body and my gums began to bleed.

DOCTOR: You noticed bruises all over and your gums were bleeding?

PATIENT: Finally, I just couldn't go to work any longer, but I didn't get better staying at home. I have an appointment to see my doctor next week and get my pills refilled, but I came to the emergency room because I couldn't go on any longer.

Up to this point, the interviewer has been open-ended, has specifically repeated words used by the patient. In response, the patient adds more symptoms. Still, specific information is needed. Each of the symptoms needs to be explored.

The patient's "tiredness" can be further clarified by questions such as:

• Tell me more about your tiredness.
• What is your tiredness like?
• When does it come on?

- How does it change throughout the day?
- How is it helped?
- What makes it worse or better?

Each of these inquires offers the patient an option. Specific inquiries will also be made about the accompanying symptoms of bruising and the bleeding gums. The patient has also mentioned seeing the doctor and getting pills refilled. These issues all need investigation by direct questioning. At any point in this sequence of questions, the patient might respond with all of the information in his own words that the physician is seeking. In fact, he might add a whole set of new and important associated data. If he has responded to each of these inquires with all the needed information, the skilled interviewer need not ask more questions. If specific information queries are kept as open as possible, the patient remains receptive to open-ended questions on other aspects of the story, rather than being forced into a question-and-answer mode.

In moving to more specific questions, the "WH" questions are frequently asked. These include who, what, when, where, why, and how the symptom occurs. The following is an example of WH questions about a complaint of pain:

1. Location. Where is the pain, where does it radiate?
2. Quality. What does it feel like?
3. Intensity. How would you rate the pain on a scale of 1 to 10?
4. Quantitative. How long does it last? How often?
5. Type of onset. How did it start?
6. Setting. What were you doing at the time of onset of the problem? How did you get through the night? When did you first see a doctor about it?
7. Aggravation and alleviation. What makes it better or worse?

With experience, the clinician will learn about a given symptom or pattern of symptoms. The decision to pursue a given topic with specific questions will be based on the potential importance for diagnosis or treatment of the specific information being sought, as well as evaluation of the patient and his responses in the interview up to that point.

Bringing Closure to the History of the Present Illness

The history of the present illness is complete when the patient has had full opportunity to tell his story and the interviewer understands the onset and progression of the symptoms. At this point it is helpful for the doctor to summarize the patient's story. The patient may agree or alter some of the details. This often produces additional information.

The interviewer can ask, "Can you think of anything else that you haven't mentioned?" The clinician is often rewarded by the patient's coming forth with entirely new data pertaining to the present illness or a new problem that needs to be addressed.

Transition from Present Illness to Past History

Before reviewing the past history, the clinician should give attention to symptoms or illnesses the patient may have that are clearly not part of the present illness but are continuing problems. Most associated illnesses receive short shrift as the clinician concentrates on the present illness. The patient may, in fact, be under treatment for one or several ongoing conditions. For example, an older man with fever, cough, wheezing, and tightness in the chest will consult a physician for diagnosis and treatment of a probable acute bronchitis, the present illness. However, he may have had increasing difficulties in urinating for some weeks, symptoms not related to his bronchitis. He is likely to express these concerns at the time he is being seen and treated for his respiratory difficulties.

Younger patients in good health may have no other current medical problems. Such patients are the exception, however. Asking the younger patient, "Do you have any other concerns about your health?" is likely to elicit worries about diet, cholesterol, weight problems, exercise, HIV status, and other health issues.

PAST MEDICAL HISTORY

Sheagren and colleagues[9] have written, "The present illness often represents a failure of medicine to recognize pre-existing conditions until they evolve into the present illness." The purpose of obtaining a careful past medical and surgical history is to elicit from the patient those pre-existing conditions that can cause or contribute to present or future illnesses.

In turning to the past history, the interviewer might ask, "How was your health before the present difficulties began?" Commonly, patients respond with "pretty good," "fair," or "not so good." Such vague responses usually reflect how the patient was feeling immediately before the present illness rather than an appraisal of his past medical and surgical history. Some patients who have been in the medical system and have been repeatedly asked about their medical histories can summarize various episodes of illness, but most patients need prompting to recall such previous medical events. It may be more helpful to begin this phase of the interview by inquiring about previous hospitalizations. Patients will remember illnesses that were serious enough to result in hospitalization, particularly if they required surgery. "Have you ever had to be hospitalized?" is a question that may provide all of the needed information about previous medical illnesses as well as operations, serious injuries, pregnancies, blood transfusions, and severe allergic reactions. It may be necessary to be more directive in eliciting the past history by asking specifically about the patient's health as a child and teenager and during successive decades to the present time (Table 3.3).

Childhood Illnesses

One need not obtain detailed information about the usual childhood diseases. It is better to ask if the patient had any unusual illnesses as a

TABLE 3.3. Components of the Past History

1. Childhood illnesses
2. Immunizations
3. Adult illnesses
4. Surgical procedures
5. Accidents and injuries
6. Allergies
7. Pregnancies

child. Patients will remember earlier serious illnesses if they interfered with school or recreational activities for a long time. A teenage girl would not forget the rash of lupus for which she always wore long sleeves in school to avoid attention. A person who had rheumatic fever as a child will always remember the long periods of confinement to bed.

Immunization History

It is important to obtain a careful immunization history since less than 50 percent of children in the United States are adequately immunized. It is essential to know whether the patient was fully immunized as a child for measles, mumps, and rubella, as well as polio, tetanus, and diphtheria. Has the woman of child-bearing age had rubella or been immunized against it?

Adult Illnesses and Surgical Procedures

As noted above, patients are more likely to recall past medical illnesses and surgical procedures if they required hospitalization. Even then, they may not remember important details, particularly if they spent time in an Intensive Care Unit. Such patients may have no memory of the reason for, duration, or course of events during their stay in a critical care unit. Such information may have to be obtained from old medical records.

The patient's report of a given diagnosis should not be accepted at face value. The previous physician may have used medical terms that were misunderstood by the patient. The interviewer will have to inquire about the details of past illnesses. For instance, patients often say they have had a heart attack, but when they are questioned, the "heart attack" may prove to have been an anxiety attack or undiagnosed chest pain. Patients with chest pain often enter the hospital fearful of a heart attack. Even though such a diagnosis was never proven, they may continue to believe the problem was a heart attack. Obtaining the old hospital records may be the only way to clearly document the diagnosis. Patients are similarly vague about the details of surgical procedures. An older woman who has undergone a hysterectomy may not know if the ovaries

or the appendix were also removed. Many patients who have had explor-
atory surgery may be uncertain about the reasons for the surgery and
may have little understanding of the surgical findings. It is important to
have access to the surgical report and the pathological findings when
there is a possibility of cancer.

Accidents and Injuries

A history of past accidents and serious injuries, particularly if there have
been several, raises a question about their cause. Repeated vehicular
accidents, or head injuries sustained in fights or assaults, may indicate
alcohol or drug abuse. Older patients who have had several falls and
fractures may have gait disturbances or osteoporosis. Serious injuries at
home account for a high incidence of morbidity and disability among
elderly people.

Allergies

The allergy history is obtained by asking about childhood or adult allergies and allergic reactions to drugs. Some patients may not make the
connection between allergy and specific allergic phenomena. For this
reason, it may be better to ask if the patient has ever had hay fever,
asthma, or hives. Food allergies are common and may be serious. All
patients should be asked if they have ever had allergic or other reactions
to drugs, either prescribed or over-the-counter. Commonly prescribed
drugs such as erythromycin or tetracycline may have caused gastrointestinal upsets that are not actually allergic in origin. Serious, sometimes
fatal reactions to medications can be prevented if these are noted in the
patient's record.

Pregnancies

It is customary to ask female patients about pregnancies and abortions.
While married women may have already spoken of a child or children,
this question could be embarrassing to sexually inactive women or to
some sexually active single women. Yet it is an important question. The

number of pregnancies, the ages at which those pregnancies took place, and their outcome are all significant data. Many women fail to distinguish between miscarriages and abortions. A careful history will serve to separate the two. Any problems occurring during pregnancy such as toxemia or maternal diabetes are important to note. Hormones taken during pregnancy and the condition of the newborn baby are important pieces of information.

Medications

The interviewer should ask the patient whether prescribed or over-the-counter drugs are taken. The patient may forget to mention over-the-counter drugs. Laxatives, cold and flu pills, sleeping aids, allergy medications, vitamins and minerals, and many other preparations may not even be regarded as drugs by the patient. Some patients may not mention herbal or homeopathic drugs because they are uncertain how the clinician might react to their use. Ask about dosage and frequency of the drugs taken. All drugs are capable of causing side effects and drug interactions. The present illness itself may be due to a reaction to a drug or even a vitamin in some cases.

Patients seeing one physician frequently fail to mention the drugs prescribed by another. A case example was given earlier of a patient who developed a bleeding peptic ulcer due to a nonsteroidal anti-inflammatory drug given to her by her physician son without the knowledge of her primary physician. When one is concerned about the medications taken, particularly if prescribed by other doctors, it may be helpful to have the patient bring all of his medications, both prescribed and over-the-counter, to the doctor's office or clinic.

SEXUAL HISTORY

Because of the intimate role of sexuality in physical and psychological health, the sexual history is an important part of the medical history. Most patients have concerns about their sexuality. Sexually active people may worry about sexually transmitted diseases. Above all, developing AIDS is a great worry, particularly among sexually active people with multiple partners and those who are homosexual or bisexual.

Many patients are concerned about sexual function that has become impaired by illness or by the medications they are taking. Depression, which often accompanies serious illness, also impairs sexual function.

Many diseases can affect sexual function. These include arthritis, neurological disorders, chronic lung and heart disease, diabetes, and many other medical and psychiatric problems.

A 63-year-old man complained to his physician of pain in the hip due to osteoarthritis. After talking about his pain, he appeared sad, and said, "I just don't feel like a man anymore." The interviewer reflected back the statement to him and the patient went on to talk about his recent trouble in obtaining an erection, how it made him feel "down, old and not like the man I used to be."

A 25-year-old man fell in love with his physical therapist while he was in a rehabilitation hospital recovering from an amputation below the knee. Before his injury he had experienced no sexual difficulty. He first became depressed after losing his leg, and even more depressed when he found his sexual function impaired with his new girlfriend, who had become his fiancée. In the interview he talked freely about his previous sexual activities while in the army. At first he was animated as he described his fiancée and how moved he had been when she gave him a watch for his birthday. Then he suddenly became tearful. The interviewer said, "She really must have touched you." He responded that he felt terrible about not being able to perform sexually as he had in the past.

Whether they are due to organic disease, personal conflicts, depression, or the effects of medication, patients are often reluctant to talk about their sexual problems. But the fact remains that most people have concerns about their sexuality that surface at different times in their lives. This is true of the sexually active as well as those who are no longer active but continue to have sexual thoughts and feelings. Sexual concerns have been shown to affect virtually all ages and sexes. While many are initially reluctant to volunteer information about their sexual activity, experts in the field of sexuality report that once the issue is raised patients welcome attention to this aspect of their lives. The patient is not the only one who has difficulty in introducing sexual topics to the interview. Many students and practicing physicians are reluctant to inquire about the patient's sexuality because of their own discomfort with the subject.

In order to pursue the subject of sexuality with the patient, it is necessary to be reasonably knowledgeable. This knowledge can be obtained from reading, lectures, and discussion groups. Examining one's feelings about teenage pregnancy, premarital sex, sexual promiscuity, unprotected sex, homosexuality, bisexuality, and sexual behavior is important since personal conflict over these issues can affect the physician's ability to discuss them and to help the patient. While many experts in this field advocate direct questioning about the patient's sexual identity and practices, there are other ways to approach this private part of the patient's life. In the course of obtaining a complete medical history the interviewer is likely to pick up clues, "windows of opportunity." The way a patient talks about his or her spouse, boyfriend, or girlfriend may signal problems. A chance remark such as, "We're not as close as we used to be," should alert the interviewer to possible sexual problems. The patient may describe the whole problem at this point.

It can be safely assumed that patients recovering from surgery may be experiencing sexual difficulties or concerns. Billings and Stoeckle[10] suggest that the interviewer use a statement of assumption as a device to introduce the subject, such as, "I suspect you have had some questions in your mind about how this surgery will affect your sexual life." Or, in the presence of chronic disease, generalizing the issue with a statement like, "Many people tell us that in situations or conditions like yours, they have some problems in functioning sexually. I wonder if you have any such concerns?" makes it easier for the patient to respond.

A 15-year-old boy, anxious about an upcoming hernia operation, anxious about surgery so close to his genitalia, is not likely to bring up the subject without prompting. Men who undergo surgery for prostatic hypertrophy or malignancy are very concerned about the effect of the procedure on their sexual functioning. Women with breast cancer worry about their sexual attractiveness after a mastectomy and even after a breast biopsy. Following a hysterectomy many women feel they have lost their sexuality. Exploring their feelings before surgery can help allay such concerns.

Patients taking drugs for the treatment of hypertension should be asked about side effects. Sexual dysfunction is commonly seen with these drugs and is always a concern to the patient when it occurs. It would be wrong, however, to assume that sexual difficulties are due to the drug without discussing the issue in a broader context. "Are you having any problems with your high blood pressure medicine?" is a better question than, "Are you have difficulty in functioning sexually since you started your medication?" The latter question is a leading one that may incorrectly target the medication as being responsible for the problem. A similar inquiry can be made to patients who abuse alcohol and drugs, as they frequently complain of loss of sexual interest or impaired sexual function.

Most women experience bladder infections at some time during their adult lives. Many associate recurrent bladder infections with their sexual activities.

A 30-year-old recently divorced graduate student complained of a recurrence of bladder infections after years of freedom from such attacks. "Have you any idea why these bladder infections have returned after so many years," the interviewer asked. The patient was quiet at first and shrugged her shoulders. The clinician went on to say, "Some patients tell us they notice a relationship between their sexual activities and bladder infections." The patient then talked about her new boyfriend and their active sexual life together after years of almost total abstinence during an unhappy marriage. She went on to say that she really knew that her bladder infections were due to her renewed sexual activity.

Frequently, patients know or suggest that there is a connection between illness and changes in their sexuality but are reluctant to talk about it early in the interview. Ill-defined complaints such as fatigue, depression, insomnia, and other vague physical and psychological symptoms should alert the interviewer to the possibility of sexual concerns. Patients recovering from a heart attack commonly worry about their sexual ability as well as the safety of resuming sexual activity and welcome a chance to talk about it.

There are many opportunities during the interview to obtain a sexual history. When inquiring about the menses, for instance, one can obtain information not only about the menarche and the regularity and frequency of periods, but also about first sexual experiences, contraception, pregnancies, and abortions. These issues may open up the whole area of sexuality. Such inquiries could be made also during the review of systems, to be described later in this chapter, or just before doing the pelvic examination. In the latter instance one would ask about premenstrual tension, painful periods, vaginal discharge, dryness of the vagina, or painful intercourse.

The developmental history provides another opportunity to obtain the sexual history as the patient talks about the changes at puberty, development of secondary sexual characteristics, early sexual experimentation, and the sexual history up to the present time. Also, it is the clinician's responsibility to inquire about sexually transmitted diseases.

In a well-conducted medical interview, the patient is likely to feel that discussing sexual matters is a natural part of the medical and psychosocial history. The interviewer tries to keep the interview as open-ended as possible, helping the patient to voice concerns that may ordinarily be difficult for him or her to talk about.

Homosexual and bisexual patients are more likely to make their sexual identity known to the clinician than they were in the past. Yet many homosexual patients will refer to hospital visitors or those at home without identifying their sex. A common error of beginning interviewers is to ask the question, "Are you married?" Until the relationship is clarified, it is wise to refer to the unidentified person with the term used by the patient, such as partner or friend. As the interview continues, the relationship will usually become clear. Gay patients may make their sexual orientation known later in the interview when better rapport has been established if the interviewer is seen as unbiased and trustworthy.

SUBSTANCE USE AND ABUSE

Obtaining the alcohol and drug history is often difficult for patient and clinician alike. While patients who drink alcohol in moderation have no reason to be defensive about it, those who drink excessively usually are. Patients who abuse alcohol tend to be guarded about it. Most substance abusers deny their problems. The subject should be explored in a supportive, nonjudgmental manner. If the physician indicates disapproval of alcohol, the patient will be even more defensive about it. The successfully recovering alcoholic or drug addict is usually straightforward in describing his past history of abuse.

There may be clues to drug or alcohol abuse as the patient relates his or her medical story. Certain symptoms suggest the possibility of alcohol abuse. Being "nervous" without any apparent reason, difficulty in sleeping, depression, and memory deficits all raise the possibility of substance abuse. Physical symptoms of unexplained abdominal pain, diarrhea, or morning vomiting may suggest use of alcohol to excess. Diminished libido, impotence, and menstrual disorders may be caused by substance abuse. A history of repeated motor vehicle accidents or other recurrent accidents should lead one to think about alcohol abuse.

A family history of alcoholism in first-degree relatives provides a natural opening to inquire about the patient's own use of alcohol. Many patients are aware of and concerned about the genetic transmission of this disorder. Some may be open to talking about their own alcohol use and that of other members of the family.

Since the alcohol-abusing patient will rarely tell the truth when asked directly about his alcohol consumption, a gradual approach may be more useful. A good approach is to begin by inquiring about the use of medications, both prescription and over-the-counter, the use of caffeine and other stimulants, smoking, and finally the use of alcohol and drugs.

The CAGE questionnaire[11] has become a widely accepted way to explore the patient's use of alcohol (Table 3.4). If the patient says he does not drink, there is no reason to use the CAGE questionnaire. However,

TABLE 3.4. The CAGE Questionnaire

Have you felt the need to Cut down on drinking?
Have you ever felt Annoyed by criticism of drinking?
Have you had Guilty feelings about drinking?
Have you ever taken a morning Eye opener?

if the patient says he drinks alcohol, this questionnaire should guide the subsequent inquiry. Before using the CAGE questionnaire, you should tell the patient that you are about to ask him a series of questions about his use of alcohol. The clinician should observe the patient's manner of response carefully. Defensiveness, evasiveness, and irritation suggest a problem with alcohol.

Alcohol abuse leads to problems with general health, accidents or injuries, legal difficulties, financial problems, problems at work, and difficulties in social relations. Thus, if responses to the CAGE questionnaire indicate that a problem with alcohol exists, these areas warrant further exploration.

In eliciting the alcohol and drug history, the interviewer must be supportive and nonjudgmental. It is important to maintain rapport with the patient during this portion of the interview. The rewards can be great. The patient may be relieved to find an understanding and supportive ear and may take the first step toward addressing a very difficult problem.

FAMILY HISTORY

In taking a family history, the interviewer seeks to obtain health information about parents, siblings, and children. Information about grandparents, aunts, uncles, and cousins may also be useful. Special interest is focused on those known inherited disorders due to the transmission of a single gene defect as well as those more common familial disorders that have environmental contributing factors.

Among the single-gene disorders are familial hypercholesterolemia, sickle cell anemia, and cystic fibrosis. More common, however, are those familial diseases with genetic susceptibility that require environmental factors for their development, such as hypertension, diabetes, coronary artery disease, rheumatoid arthritis, and colon and breast cancer. A good opening question in eliciting the family history is, "Are there any illnesses that run in your family?"

Either a tabular format or a pedigree diagram (genogram) is used in recording the family history. The tabular format is simply a list:

- Maternal grandmother died at the age of 78, stroke.
- Maternal grandfather died at the age of 61, pneumonia.
- Paternal grandmother died at the age of 74, cause unknown.
- Paternal grandfather died at the age of 57, diabetes, coronary thrombosis.
- Mother died at the age of 66, lymphoma.
- Father died at the age of 66, coronary thrombosis.
- One brother died at the age of 52, coronary thrombosis.
- One brother alive and well at 69, history of prostatic cancer.
- Two sons, ages 48 and 40, living and well.

When concerned about hereditary diseases in particular, a pedigree diagram may be helpful. Such a pedigree diagram is shown in Figure 3.1.

A family history also includes the current health history of parents, siblings, and other family members. Ask patients with febrile illnesses if there is anyone else sick at home. When one suspects the patient has been exposed to toxic substances at home, it is important to know if other family members have similar symptoms.

The family history may reveal problems in family relations and family conflicts. Also, since most patients are keenly aware of the cause and age of death of their parents and siblings, they may be worried that they will die of the same disease and about at the same age. Reviewing the family history with the patient can bring out hidden concerns about their own mortality. It may identify illnesses that can be prevented by altering health-related behavior.

REVIEW OF SYSTEMS

A clinician who proceeds in the manner described thus far is likely to uncover most of the relevant data about the patient's health. However, important information might still go undetected. The review of systems, organ system by organ system, is designed to reduce the likelihood of missing essential data. The necessity for pursuing a detailed survey is usually determined by the complexity of the present illness. A young

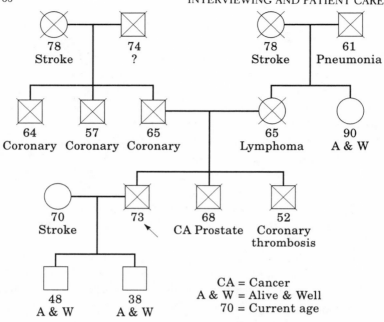

FIGURE 3.1. Pedigree Diagram. In a pedigree diagram, males are represented by squares and females by circles. A diagonal line through a symbol indicates that the person has died. Siblings are arranged from left to right in order of birth with the first-born (eldest) sibling on the far left. A number within or below the circle or square represents the person's age or age at death. The patient is designated with an arrow.

patient with an acute illness of only a few days' duration who states he has always been healthy is less likely to have involvement of several organ systems than an older patient with a chronic disease. The review of systems increases the probability that the history is complete.

Information already obtained from the patient will also guide the review of systems. The patient with a strong family history of early-onset coronary artery disease who has not complained of cardiac symptoms should nonetheless be questioned about risk factors for heart disease including hypertension, elevated cholesterol, and symptoms of chest pain. Similarly, the heavy cigarette smoker should be queried about shortness of breath, cough, and sputum to rule out pulmonary disease.

In pursuing the systems review, one should ask a general question pertaining to a given organ system. If the patient replies in the negative or gives only inconsequential information, the interviewer may move on. On the other hand, if the patient gives a positive response, the interviewer narrows the questions to obtain specific information (Table 3.5).

The systems review is best done during the course of the physical examination. When the physician is examining a particular part of the body, questions appropriate to that region or organ system are asked. While examining the eyes, one can ask the question, "Do you have any problems with your vision?" Before examining the abdomen, one might ask if there has been any difficulty with the stomach or bowel.

There are advantages in doing the system review while examining the patient. Talking with the patient while he is being examined lessens his anxiety. Many patients are fearful of what the doctor might find. They

TABLE 3.5. System Review

---

a. Systemic

Any general symptoms such as fever, weight loss, fatigue, nausea, poor appetite?

b. Skin

Any skin problems? Sores? Rashes? Growths? Itching? Changes in the hair or nails? Dryness?

c. Eyes

Any changes in vision? Pain? Redness? Discharge? Double vision? Watery eyes?

d. Ears

How are the ears and hearing? Running ears? Poor hearing? Ringing ears?

e. Nose

How are your nose and sinuses? Stuffy nose? Discharge? Bleeding? Unusual odors?

f. Mouth

Any problems with your mouth? Sores? Bad taste? Sore tongue? Gum trouble?

(continued)

TABLE 3.5. System Review (*continued*)

g. Throat and Neck
    Any problems with your throat and neck? Sore throat? Hoarseness? Swelling? Swallowing?

h. Breasts
    Any problems with your breasts? Lumps? Nipple discharge? Bleeding? Swelling? Tenderness?

i. Pulmonary
    Any problems with your lungs or breathing? Cough? Sputum? Bloody sputum? Pain in the chest upon taking a deep breath, shortness of breath?

j. Cardiovascular
    Do you have any problems with your heart? Chest pain? Shortness of breath? Palpitations? Cough? Swelling of your ankles? Trouble lying flat in bed at night? Fatigue?

k. Gastrointestinal
    How is your digestion? Any changes in your appetite? Nausea? Vomiting? Diarrhea? Constipation? Change in your bowel habits? Bleeding from the rectum? Hemorrhoids?

l. Genitourinary-male
    Any problems with your kidneys or urination? Painful urination? Frequency? Urgency? Nocturia? Bloody or cloudy urine? Trouble starting or stopping?

m. Genitourinary-female
    Number of pregnancies? Abortions? Miscarriages? Any menstrual problems? Last menstrual period? Vaginal bleeding? Vaginal discharge? Cessation of periods? Hot flashes? Vaginal itching?

n. Endocrine
    Any problems with your endocrine glands? Feeling hot or cold? Fatigue? Changes in the skin or hair? Frequent urination? Fatigue?

o. Musculoskeletal
    Do you have any problems with your bones or joints? Joint or muscle pain? Stiffness? Limitation of motion?

p. Peripheral nervous system
    Numbness? Weakness? Pins and needles sensation?

become anxious and uncomfortable if the examiner concentrates on the physical exam without saying a word. Also, there is a feeling that the communication established during the course of the interview has been suspended. Continuing with some dialogue also prods the patient's memory about symptoms relating to the particular organ being examined.

It is best to ask questions before examining a particular area. In examining the heart, for example, if the clinician asks a question about the heart after listening with the stethoscope, the patient is often fearful that something wrong has been discovered. Then it becomes necessary to allay his or her unnecessary concern.

INTERVIEWING DURING THE PHYSICAL EXAMINATION

In most cases patients expect the physician to examine them following the interview. The degree of thoroughness of the physical exam varies according to the clinical problem and the physician's primary interests. The physical exam also can become an extension of the interview. The "laying on of hands" does affect the patient-doctor relationship. During or after the examination a change often takes place in the level of communication between doctor and patient.

A 65-year-old woman, a Christian Scientist, was discovered to have breast cancer several weeks earlier by her gynecologist. These studies had been done while her husband was away on a business trip. Her eldest daughter was staying with her while her husband was away, and she had insisted that her mother have a long overdue mammogram. The mammogram findings were suspicious and led to a needle biopsy that revealed a malignancy. A family conference took place after the husband's return, but the patient could not be convinced of the need for medical care. Instead, she sought the help of the Christian Science practitioner. The practitioner advised her to have at least a complete physical examination before refusing surgery. During the interview preceding the physical examination, the patient was wary, formal, closed, and had no rapport with the physician. As the physical examination was coming to a close, there was a noticeable change in the patient's appearance and behavior. She appeared to relax, no longer holding herself so rigidly. Then she gradually began to tell the story of what she had gone through since the discovery of the lump—her fear of cancer and her fear of dying. She spoke of the immense conflict she was having between following her religious beliefs and accepting surgery. Finally, she spoke of what a relief it was to be able to talk about it.

Toward the end of the physical examination, patients frequently raise issues of a personal nature not discussed during the initial interview. It is a time when the patient may feel more comfortable talking about the real reason for the visit to the physician. Today, patients often ask, "Do you think I should have an AIDS test?" They may wait through the entire medical history before raising their deepest concerns.

CONCLUSION

The medical history is the most important part of the clinician's evaluation of a patient's problems. Though some specialists may focus on a limited component of the history, all physicians must develop the skills of obtaining a complete history. Even in a focused interview, it is important to be aware of the patient's total health status in order to complete a proper evaluation. The amount of attention given to each component varies with every patient and each illness. While all aspects of the medical history are not investigated in every patient visit, it is important that the clinician be familiar with all of them.

REFERENCES

1. Balint, M., *The Doctor, His Patient and the Illness*. New York: International University Press, 1957.
2. Barsky, Arthur J., "Hidden Reasons Some Patients Visit Doctors," *Annals of Internal Medicine*, 94:492–498, 1981.
3. Burack, Robert C., and Robert R. Carpenter, "The Predictive Value of the Presenting Complaint," *The Journal of Family Practice*, 16, 4:749–754, 1983.

4. Beckman, Howard B., and Richard D. Frankel, "The Effect of Physician Behavior on the Collection of Data," *Annals of Internal Medicine*, 101:692–696, 1984.

5. Branch, William T., and Tariq K. Malik, "Using Windows of Opportunity in Brief Interviews to Understand Patients' Concerns," *Journal of the American Medical Association*, 269, 13:1667–1668, 1993.

6. Smith, Robert C., and Ruth B. Hoppe, "The Patient's Story: Integrating the Patient- and Physician-Centered Approaches to Interviewing," *Annals of Internal Medicine*, 115, 6:470–477, 1991.

7. Leigh, Hoyle, and Morton F. Reiser, *The Patient: Biological, Psychological, and Social Dimensions of Medical Practice*. New York: Plenum Medical Book Company, 1980.

8. Payne, S. L., *The Art of Asking Questions*. Princeton, N.J.: Princeton University Press, 1951.

9. Sheagren, John N., Andrew J. Zweifler, and James O. Woolliscroft, "The Present Medical Database Needs Reorganization," *Archives Internal Medicine*, 150:2014–2015, 1990.

10. Billings, J. Andrew, and John D. Stoeckle, *The Clinical Encounter*. Chicago: Year Book Medical Publishers, 1989.

11. Ewing, J. A., "Detecting Alcoholism, The CAGE Questionnaire," *Journal of American Medical Association*, 252:1905, 1984.

4

INTERVIEWING PATIENTS UNDER SPECIAL CIRCUMSTANCES

KEY POINTS

1. With non-English speaking patients precautions must be taken to ensure a reasonably accurate translation.
2. Persons from other cultures may have difficulty with open-ended interviewing and may require more directive questioning.
3. Interviewing a mildly cognitively imparied patient or a psychotic patient may be difficult, and a mental status examination may be in order.
4. The mental status examination requires attention to appearance and behavior, speech, mood, thought content or preoccupations, orientation, and cognition.
5. Special arrangements are needed for blind patients.
6. Specifically focused interviews are needed in the emergency room and the ICU, where both patient and family often must be interviewed.

In the preceding chapters we discussed the model and techniques that are most useful in gathering the data necessary for diagnosis and treatment and in establishing a positive doctor-patient relationship. Their application calls for flexibility, however. Conditions under which clinical interviews take place vary. They change with the setting, time constraints and the type of patient. Appropriate modifications are called for with patients from other cultures, those who require an interpreter, demented patients, psychotic patients, and patients who are visually or hearing impaired. Settings such as special care units and medical or surgical subspecialty clinics or offices dictate changes in approach. Time constraints in managed care and other situations may call for adjusting the interview style and focusing on immediate problems. In this chapter we will discuss these applications of patient-centered interviewing principles.

CROSS-CULTURAL CONSIDERATIONS

When a patient does not speak English and it is necessary to use an interpreter, the clinician must take certain precautions to ensure an accurate account. This is not too difficult when a professional interpreter is available. Otherwise, one must use nonprofessional, bilingual individuals who are available. The least satisfactory interpreters are family members, as they have the greatest difficulty in carrying out the task in the manner outlined below.

Whether the interpreter is a professional, a staff member who is conveniently present and is bilingual or, as a last resort, a family member, it is important to address the patient directly. A common error is addressing questions to the interpreter, in effect requesting the interpreter to obtain certain information. This delegates the interviewing task to someone who is rarely a trained interviewer. The following procedures should be utilized:

1. Interview the nonprofessional interpreter briefly to ascertain his or her fluency in English. It is not helpful to use a person who is marginally fluent in English. If a nonprofessional interpreter is being used, the clinician should instruct the volunteer about how the interview will proceed.
2. Address all questions to the patient as though the patient speaks English. Use simple language and avoid medical or clinical terms

    that may be difficult for the interpreter to translate or for the patient to understand.

3. Instruct the interpreter to translate exactly what you have said. If the interpreter states that there is no exact equivalent in the other language, rephrase the question in simpler terms.

4. The patient's response must be translated as accurately as possible, allowing for colloquialisms. The interpreter should not try to explain "what the patient means," paraphrase, omit details, or add his own thoughts. This is particularly difficult when a family member must be used.

5. Look at the patient, not the interpreter or the chart. Observe the patient's facial expressions and such movements and behavior as posture, touching of body parts, and gestures.

An open-ended interview style is possible with an interpreter if these principles are followed. However, such an interview style may be less successful with patients from other cultures than with native-born, English-speaking patients. This is especially the case when there is a disparity between the socioeconomic status of the patient and that of the clinician. Many persons of lower socioeconomic status from Asian or Latin cultures view the doctor or other health professional as an authority to whom deference and compliance are due. They may have difficulty giving a spontaneous, minimally guided account. The result is that the interviewer may have to use more directive questioning earlier in the interview than with other patients.

Nilchaikovit and co-authors described Asian and American differences in illness behavior, interactions with physicians, communication style, and expression of emotion.[1] American patients tend to be verbal, open, direct, and expressive. Asian patients tend to be quiet and indirect and to value serenity, stoicism, and suppression of negative emotion. The predominant form of the physician-patient relationship in the United States according to these authors, is a contractual agreement in which the patient's participation is of crucial importance. By contrast, Indochinese immigrants, for example, see physicians as authority figures endowed with knowledge, experience, and wisdom. Patients are expected to show respect and deference for the physician's authority and to feel grateful for his help. Western doctors may feel frustrated when interviewing Asian patients because they tend to be quiet and passive, rarely volunteer details, understate their problems, and seldom express their feelings. Thus, the physician must be more active and more directive in seeking the information necessary for diagnosis and treatment.

There have been many studies of cultural differences in the way pain is described. Zborowski[2] and Zola[3,4] published early studies of the response to pain in American patients of Old American, Jewish, Irish, and Italian origin. Zborowski described Jewish and Italian patients as emphasizing or "playing up" their perception of pain while Old American and Irish patients tended to deemphasize or "play down" pain and were more apt to differentiate between slight, severe, and very severe pain. Zola, who studied lower-class Italians, Irish, and Anglo-Saxons seeking aid at a large urban hospital outpatient department, found that patients of Italian descent reported pain more frequently than did patients of Irish or Anglo-Saxon descent and were more often labeled "psychiatric problems" by their physicians despite a lack of evidence that psychiatric disorders were more common among them. A recent study of patients coming to the same clinic 20 years later indicated that there were now age differences in this behavior. Italian patients over 60 years of age behaved as described by Zola, but younger patients were much less likely to do so.[5]

When an interpreter has translated the patient's description of symptoms such as pain or physiological changes, it is well to check your understanding by summarizing and inviting correction or additional details. A statement like, "Tell me if I understand what you said," followed by repeating what you believe the patient to have said is useful. Then add, "Is that right?" or, "Or is there something else you were telling me?"[6]

THE COGNITIVELY IMPAIRED PATIENT

A difficult situation for the clinician is the interview of a patient with mild cognitive impairment. To complicate matters, many such patients have a repertoire of socially appropriate statements including greetings and standard remarks. They may not even know who you are or why they are being interviewed yet may behave pleasantly and answer queries with misleadingly ambiguous but seemingly responsive statements. Some patients, especially those whose cognitive impairment is related to alcohol abuse, may fabricate experiences. This is called *confabulation*. If these confabulations are not clearly improbable, they can be convincing enough to be mistaken for actual memories.

In elderly patients with subtle signs of early dementia, a mental status evaluation is especially important, though it is part of any diagnostic interview. The mental status examination is part of the fabric of interviewing and is carried out through careful observation during the course of the interview. Everything about an individual—general appearance, grooming, dress, behavior, and language—gives clues to possible impairment of cognition.[7]

The assessment of mental status goes on throughout the period of time that the clinician and patient are together. In many, if not most, cases very few specific inquiries need be made since it can be easily ascertained whether or not the basic areas of mental functioning are within normal limits. This means, however, that the examiner has had these areas of mental functioning in mind throughout the interview. The examiner listens to what the patient says and how he says it. If this yields evidence that the patient's mental status needs close scrutiny, the physician can make appropriate inquiries.

Attention should be paid to the following areas: appearance and behavior, speech, mood, thought content or preoccupations, orientation in time and space, and cognition. Posture or carriage, dress, facial expression, and attitude can reflect mood states such as sadness, anxiety, bewilderment, distrust, or hostility. Tone of voice, inflection, and volume of speech will also give clues to the patient's mood state. If the patient does not tell you spontaneously, one should ask how he feels. A confrontation about observed behavior indicating sadness, apprehension, or withdrawal may promote a discussion of depression or other feelings. Hints about suicidal tendencies should be followed up and thoroughly explored. One should attempt to assess how realistic the patient's preoccupations appear to be.

When orientation and cognition are severely impaired, it is usually obvious. More subtle signs may include carelessness in dressing, difficulty in giving dates of onset or duration of symptoms, or a bewildered look. In doubtful cases, a simple cognitive screening examination can be done without unduly affronting the patient, provided that it is introduced in a tactful way.

A good beginning is to say, "I would like to ask you a few questions. They may seem a little silly or obvious, and they may be very easy to answer, though some may be very hard. However, bear with me as I need this information in order to help you." When the patient has nodded or verbally given assent, one can then ask questions designed to assess basic cognitive status.

Orientation can be assessed by asking: What day of the week is this? What month? What day of the month? What year? To test immediate recall, ask the patient to repeat three numbers and then ask him to say them backwards. If the patient repeats them accurately, give him four numbers. Then for somewhat delayed recall, ask the patient to count one through ten out loud before repeating three numbers that you have just given him. A few simple arithmetic questions such as adding or subtracting two numbers can be posed. Also ask the patient to say the days of the week backwards, beginning with Sunday. Give the patient four unrelated words such as "chair, car, flower, twenty-six," and instruct him to repeat them after you and remember them as they will be asked for in a few minutes. Then ask a few other questions and about three or four minutes later ask for the four words. This is a test of delayed recall.

If the patient has difficulty with any of these tasks, a more detailed cognitive examination is indicated, and this is best carried out by a psychiatrist or clinical psychologist.

THE PSYCHOTIC PATIENT

Psychiatric consultation is also indicated when the interviewer finds that he cannot follow the patient's account, that it doesn't seem to make sense or flits from topic to topic without an obvious connection between them.

This can indicate a mood disorder or schizophrenia. When the patient's account seems incomprehensible or very scattered, a psychiatric consultation is in order.

VISUALLY IMPAIRED PATIENTS

We tend to underestimate the limitations on communication imposed by blindness because we can talk with the blind freely. Many blind people are articulate conversationalists. The sighted individual may not recognize that the whole range of visual cues in conversation is denied the visually impaired or blind person. Instead, persons with marked visual impairments use a highly developed compensatory strategy in interpreting the range of sounds that are part of the verbal exchange. From such things as tone of voice and very slight auditory cues, they can gauge the mood, character, style, and attitudes of the other person. Tone of voice, sounds of body movements, clearing the throat, laughter, and a host of other cues of which sighted persons are only marginally aware are detected and interpreted with great acuity. These may not conform to the picture that a sighted person would get from the encounter. In interviews there is thus a smaller and more fragile margin for misunderstanding, even as the relationship between patient and interviewer develops.

One should tell the visually impaired person something about the surroundings into which he is being taken, whether it is an examining room, office, or other setting. Inform the patient of the approximate size and shape of the room, where the major items of furniture are located, and the locations of entrances, curtains, and so forth. Other persons present, if any, and their location should be identified at the outset. The other people present might say a few words to establish their voice pattern for the patient. If you move around the room, describe what you are doing in a brief matter-of-fact way. Give the patient the opportunity to ask questions about the environment before the interview begins.

Above all, avoid changing your usual conversational behavior. Do not increase the volume of your speech or change its normal pace, overarticulating or speaking in short and simplifed sentences. Surprisingly, blind people are often dealt with in this way. They find it highly offensive.

THE HEARING-IMPAIRED PATIENT

Impaired hearing is common in older patients. When such patients are not sufficiently impaired to warrant a hearing aid, communication can be unsatisfying for both patient and interviewer. This is especially true in hospital or clinic settings where there is a good deal of background noise. Even in a relatively quiet room, a soft-spoken interviewer may be imperfectly heard by such patients. Women's voices, often soft and not well projected, may be particularly difficult for them to hear.

When one becomes aware of a problem in communicating, it is common for the interviewer to raise his voice briefly and then to resume his or her usual pattern of speech, once again becoming marginally audible. The use of a portable hearing augmentation device such as those available in theatres can be of great value to the hearing-impaired patient.

Patients who have hearing aids should be encouraged to use them as they may not be wearing them at the moment. It may be wise to defer the interview until the hearing aid is available. Many hearing-impaired patients are able to lip-read. The interviewer should sit in a well-lighted location where his face is easily seen and should face the patient while speaking. Articulate normally; do not overarticulate as this is more difficult for the patient to interpret than normal speech. Speak at a moderate, even pace.

However, lipreading is not a reliable method of communication for most patients. According to Lotke,[8] the average profoundly deaf lipreader understands approximately one-third of what is said to him. Persons with less impairment generally have better success at lipreading because they can use the parts of sound they hear to supplement what they see on the speaker's lips. This is especially true for those who have lost their hearing over time. The congenitally deaf often know American Sign Language. For them a professional ASL interpreter makes the interview far more successful.

THE EMERGENCY ROOM

In the emergency room, modifications of interviewing style are often necessary.

For many of the patients who come to the emergency room, the interviewing task is much the same as in the office or medical clinic. Depending on the patient's condition, however, the physician working in the emergency room must shift back and forth between open-ended, patient-centered interviewing and a directive, physician-centered style. In true emergency situations, interviews are focused on the immediate problem. Often patients are in pain. They may have impaired consciousness, be extremely anxious, or be unable to speak at all. It is usually helpful if family members or others who can give a history of the events leading to the patient's coming to the emergency room are present.

There is usually very little privacy in the emergency room, if any. To the extent that it is possible, one should try to preserve the patient's privacy and maintain a gentle and supportive manner even though conducting a highly focused interview.

SPECIAL CARE UNITS (ICU AND CCU)

Patients seen in Coronary Care Units or Intensive Care Units may have arrived from the emergency room or from special diagnostic areas where cardiac catheterization or other diagnostic procedures have been performed. In CCU some are awaiting such studies. ICU patients may be unable to communicate. All are anxious. When patients are in CCU or ICU, therefore, it is essential that the interview remain open-ended, patient-centered, and supportive. The patient may or may not deny anxiety, but even if not verbalized, the behavioral signs of anxiety will almost always be discernible. It is important to give those patients who can the opportunity to express this anxiety, to offer appropriate support, and to convey understanding of the depth of their anxiety.

THE MEDICAL AND SURGICAL SUBSPECIALIST

Health care workers vary widely in their specific requirements for information from and about the patient. Primary care physicians such as internists, pediatricians, and family practitioners interview patients at length when conditions permit. Consulting specialists and subspecialists tend to limit their interview to specific data about the onset and further development of the presenting symptoms. When the subspecialist sees little need for interview data, a doctor-patient relationship of depth and strength usually does not develop. While it is unnecessary for specialists and subspecialists to obtain for themselves the general information about the patient that is characteristically obtained by a primary physician, since much of this is available from the referring doctor, it is inexcusable to do no interviewing other than to inquire about the history of the onset and development of the presenting symptoms. The open-ended style of interviewing is useful even when the focus of the interviewer is a skin lesion or upper respiratory symptom. Even in the brief time allotted for such examinations, one can begin with an open-ended question and explore some of the concurrent problems that the patient may have.

A self-confident 43-year-old professional woman who was successful in her field was referred to a pulmonologist because of a particularly stubborn lung infection that had not responded to treatment. The specialist was able to identify the causal organism, and after prescribing a regimen of antibiotics, he obtained laboratory evidence that the infection was gone. Nonetheless, the patient continued to have the same symptoms. Finally, phoning the referring internist to express his puzzlement over the continuation of these symptoms, the pulmonologist learned for the first time that the patient was involved in an extremely unhappy and stressful marriage and was struggling with the decision about separating from her husband. She had never mentioned this to the specialist as his interviews were focused and did not allow her the opportunity to talk about her marital problems.

CONCLUSION

The principles of open-ended interviewing require some modification with special types of patients or under special circumstances. These include non-English speaking patients, patients from other cultures, patients with impaired cognitive function, visually impaired patients, the hearing-impaired, and patients interviewed in the emergency room, the ICU, and the office of the subspecialist. To the extent possible, however, principles of open-ended interviewing should be utilized within the limitations imposed by these special circumstances.

REFERENCES

1. Nilchaikovit, T., J. M. Hill, and J. C. Holland, "The Effects of Culture on Illness Behavior and Medical Care; Asian and American Differences," *General Hospital Psychiatry*, 15:41–50, 1993.
2. Zborowski, M., *People in Pain*. San Francisco: Jossey-Bass, 1969.
3. Zola, I. K., "Problems of Communications, Diagnosis and Patient Care: The Interplay of Patient, Physician and Clinic Organization," *Journal of Medical Education*, 38:829, 1963.
4. Zola, I. K., "Culture and Symptoms: An Analysis of Patients' Presenting Complaints," *American Sociological Review*, 31:615, 1966.
5. Koopman, C., S. Eisenthal, and J. D. Stoeckle, "Ethnicity in the Reported Pain, Emotional Distress and Requests of Medical Outpatients," *Social Science and Medicine*, 18:487–490, 1984.
6. Putsch, R. W., "Cross-Cultural Communication. The Special Case of Interpreters in Health Care," *Journal of the American Medical Association*, 254:3344–3348, 1985.

7. Jones, T. V., and M. E. Williams, "Rethinking the Approach to Evaluating Mental Functioning of Older Persons. The Value of Careful Observations," *Journal of the American Geriatric Society*, 36:1128–1134, 1988.

8. Litke, M., "She Won't Look at Me," *Annals of Internal Medicine*, 123:54–57, 1995.

5

EMOTIONAL RESPONSES TO PATIENTS AND TO ILLNESS

KEY POINTS

1. Certain attributes and behaviors of the patient can produce relatively strong reactions in the interviewer that interfere with the interviewing task.
2. The patient's appearance may prejudice the clinician.
3. Behavior that is intimidating, controlling, demanding, excessively flattering, defensive, remote, hostile, or complaining can trigger negative responses from the interviewer, which will interfere with the conduct of the interview.
4. The interviewer must always keep his role clearly in mind and look past the behavior to the factors causing it.
5. The interviewer's behavior may also elicit undesirable reactions from the patient that complicate the interviewing task.

All patients evoke an emotional response in the clinician. We like some patients better than others. Some elicit strong feelings that can range from attraction to repugnance. Fortunately, however, our reaction to most patients is not so intense. Nonetheless, clinicians are never neutral in their feelings toward their patients.

One need not feel guilty if one's reaction to a given patient is negative. This is not "bad" in itself. But it is necessary to be aware of it and to cope with it—to look beyond one's emotional response and whatever evoked it. In fact, such a reaction to a patient may signal behavior that is relevant to his or her problems. At such times it especially important to keep one's role with the patient clearly in focus: The patient is there for help. The clinician is there to provide that help, either directly or as the first step in the diagnostic and treatment process. The student, too, is part of that process.

In this chapter we address attitudes and behaviors of patients that may produce an emotional response in the clinician and some typical reactions. The factors to be considered are the patient's appearance and behavior; the effect of differences in age, gender, and sexual orientation; differences in culture, ethnicity, and belief systems between the patient and the clinician; and the effects of the clinician's personal experiences with illness in himself and in his family members. We will also discuss patient responses to illness and to the interviewer that can evoke reactions from the clinician.

RESPONSES OF THE CLINICIAN

Appearance

We commonly make judgments about others based on their appearance, including dress and grooming. Though a natural tendency, this can pose a serious impediment to the interview and to the clinician-patient relationship. Students, as well as seasoned clinicians, often feel distaste when confronted with a patient who is unkempt, unwashed, smelly, or otherwise gives evidence of poor personal hygiene. In a teaching exercise at the University of Southern California School of Medicine Introduction to Clinical Medicine program, students are shown videotaped excerpts of interviews with such patients (among others). They are then asked how they responded to the patient. Almost uniformly the students have expressed distaste ranging from mild to strong dislike. Other patients whose appearance may produce a negative response, especially in students, are the obese, the physically unattractive, and those whose dress or grooming is markedly unconventional.

The clinician must look beyond the patient's superficial characteristics. For one thing, they can be misleading. Conversely, they may, and often do, reflect the problems that have led the patient to seek medical attention. One's response to appearance and behavior may have important diagnostic significance. The responsible clinician admits his feelings to himself, then puts them in perspective and gets to the task at hand, the diagnostic medical interview.

A 29-year-old black male was initially seen lying on the hospital bed in an unconventional manner. As the student entered the ward to conduct the interview, the resident and charge nurse indicated by facial expression and manner that they considered him to be a troublesome patient. As the student approached the bed, she noted that he was lying in the prone position, his left foot at the head of the bed on a pillow and his head at the foot of the bed. He had an angry, disgruntled look on his face. He was a rather muscular male whose hair was braided in a style known as "dreadlocks." He was unshaven, shirtless, and did not move, nor did his facial expression change when the student approached. The student, a rather sensitive and usually supportive young woman, began the interview in open-ended fashion and listened supportively, facilitating his account. As he spoke, his facial expression softened and he became increasingly communicative. The student learned that he was employed as the manager of a cleaning establishment, that he was quite articulate, and that he knew a great deal about his diabetic condition. He had attended patient education programs having to do with diabetes, checked his blood sugar four times a day, and injected insulin, keeping himself in perfect diabetic control. He understood his condition well and was somewhat disgruntled about the inflexibility of the hospital routine and the negative response that he was eliciting from health care personnel on the ward, which was apparently due to his appearance. His foot was on the pillow because he had a painful abscess, a complication of diabetes. After the interview, the student remarked to the instructor, "He is the sort of patient that I would like to be able to take care of," admitting that she had initially been somewhat put off by his appearance.

Equally significant impediments can hamper the relationship between the interviewer and the patient who is attractive to him. It is natural to respond positively to such patients and to give behavioral evidence of this response. This can create problems not only in the initial interview but also in later encounters with that patient. If the clinician does not take this possibility into account, he is likely to be less critically aware of the problems that stem from becoming overly involved emotionally. The role of the physician is both participant and observer. While one can be moved by a patient's behavior and story, one must strive to maintain a degree of detachment sufficient to permit careful observation. This is essential to both diagnosis and treatment. When the clinician is attracted to the patient, it is difficult to maintain that degree of detachment. This can be an especially taxing task if the patient is flirtatious or sexually attractive to the clinician.

When the clinician-interviewer feels physically attracted to the patient, this is a danger signal. During the initial interview, the clinician must be careful to maintain appropriate professional behavior with the patient. After the initial interview, if there is to be continuing professional contact with that patient, some soul-searching is needed. Ask yourself, "Will I be able to maintain an appropriate professional role without having to struggle with intrusive feelings of sexual attraction?" If the answer is no, arrange to have another person replace you on the medical team.

Behavior

A particular problem for the student clinician is the intimidating and controlling patient, who is usually older than the student. Such a patient is likely to evoke the feelings of insecurity with which every student must cope. A typical reaction of beginning interviewers is to withdraw and avoid exploring aspects of the patient's history that could be embarrassing. As a result, important data may be missed. Patients who behave in a self-assured, patronizing manner evoke a negative response and may inhibit the student-clinician from exploring important issues.

In a group exercise students were shown a videotape in which the patient being interviewed was just such an intimidating and controlling person. The patient, a 49-year-old mechanic, was dressed in a jacket and necktie and displayed a condescending manner as he described some six back operations performed by various orthopedic surgeons at his insistence. The operations had not succeeded in alleviating his symptoms. He referred to the surgeons as highly regarded in the past but now over the hill, and he contrasted their shabby treatment of patients with his own highly responsible behavior toward clients. He often interrupted the student-interviewer in the middle of a question or comment and told his own story in his own way, ignoring the particular areas that the student was attempting to explore. When asked if they would like to interview such a patient, all the students said no. They were intimidated by him even on a videotape. Of course, this same patient had probably intimidated all six of the surgeons so that they performed the unsuccessful and perhaps unnecessary operations.

A particularly trying type of patient is the hostile, belligerent, and uncooperative person, who is often critical of doctors. It is difficult to avoid responding in kind. If a patient is particularly challenging, the clinician may find himself drawn into an argument or exchange of hostile remarks. When that happens, the clinician has abandoned his role and his usefulness to the patient is severely compromised. Such encounters are indeed a trial of patience for the clinician, who must curb natural impulses and remain aware that the patient's behavior is "grist for the mill." In short, this behavior is probably a symptom of emotional difficulties, or it may be a response to chronic pain or disappointments in previous health care experiences. The most effective approach to such a patient is to begin supportive inquiries into the behavior and its origins. A good opening into such an inquiry is the simple comment, "I can't help but notice that you seem angry."

There are times when the interviewer finds himself the target of an irrational angry outburst seemingly unconnected with him. Anger may be displaced from an unavailable target (spouse or employer for example) or from an immediately preceding situation in which the patient did not have the opportunity to express his angry response. For example, a receptionist may have handled the patient in a cold and abrupt manner and turned away without allowing him a chance to voice his anger. In the hospital a patient may have been treated insensitively shortly before by a technician, nurse, or orderly. A little time will permit the anger to subside. A comment like, "I find it puzzling that you are angry with me," may uncover the true source of the anger.

Students sometimes become upset when they encounter an apparently irrational angry response from a patient they are about to interview. Sometimes the patient ascribes the anger to the fact that it is a student who is about to interview or examine him. This calls for an examination of the patient's anger with the student. A confrontation is the best way to proceed. "You sound very angry," focuses the interview on the patient's behavior and permits the likely removal of that barrier to a successful interview by a discussion of the patient's feelings. It sometimes happens that a patient or family member may refuse to be interviewed by a student. At that point, it is best to bow out gracefully and call for help from a staff member, supervisor, or resident physician.

Of course, there are also times when the clinician has provoked the anger himself. Brusqueness, sarcasm, moralistic comments, or attitudes of superiority easily provoke anger. Hopefully, this is a matter of thoughtlessness or haste and not the doctor's customary behavior. Too often doctors interview hurriedly because of time pressure. One should always examine one's own behavior before ascribing anger to some difficulty or personality trait of the patient. If the clinician encounters anger from many patients, he should look for a source in his own behavior with patients.

The patient who is friendly, respectful, polite, and complimentary is always more warmly received by the clinician. But there are pitfalls with such a patient, too. Objectivity becomes more difficult to maintain when such politeness and respectfulness reaches the point of flattery; if it is overdone, the physician may respond with distaste or annoyance.

Demanding patients are very likely to evoke annoyance. The whining patient who complains excessively usually provokes a negative response. In continuing care of such a patient, the clinician may discount or pay little attention to the ongoing litany of complaints and may thus miss an important complaint or symptom that signals a serious pathological condition.

The stoic patient is likely to be one who utilizes denial excessively and who does not complain when, in fact, a complaint would be appropriate. Clinicians often welcome such patients as they do not make demands. Therein lies the pitfall. The clinician who does not remain alert to the significance of such behavior and does not pursue minor clues may fail to obtain significant diagnostic information.

Clinicians almost universally find it distasteful to work with defensive, distant, or cold patients. They may react by ending the interview as quickly as possible, to the detriment of the information-gathering task.

The complaining patient is often a difficult one for those clinicians who value stoic or uncomplaining behavior.

> A 53-year-old woman was interviewed by a first-year medical student. She complained bitterly of post-operative pain following a total knee replacement. Before surgery, she had experienced increasing pain in the arthritic knee and had been forced to limit her activities. In telling the patient's story to a group of his peers, the student was quite critical of her "bellyaching" about a "little pain." When asked why he was unsympathetic, he declared, "She's not like my mother who has been in a wheelchair for 20 years with rheumatoid arthritis, raised four sons, and never complained once about her pain or disability."

This student was proud of his mother for coping well with a severe, progressive and debilitating disease. But he was so amazed by the patient's inability to deal with pain in a similar way that he could not appreciate her distress and felt no empathy for her.

Belief Systems

On occasion, a patient may express attitudes or beliefs that are unacceptable to the interviewer, such as political or religious opinions the interviewer regards as extreme, distasteful, or bigoted. The temptation to reason or argue with such a patient must be firmly resisted.

Patients with religious beliefs differing from those of the interviewer may arouse feelings that interfere with effective listening. The following history is an example of this:

> A student-physician was interviewing a 52-year-old waitress who was hospitalized because of severe back pain. A bone scan had indicated metastatic cancer. The site of the primary cancer was thought to be a recently discovered lump in her breast. The patient had not yet been told the diagnosis. At the time of the interview she was concerned about obtaining

relief from her back pain. In talking about her work as a waitress she described her difficulty during a period of economic recession in finding a job. She said she would pray "to the Lord" to help her find work. She had always found work and ascribed this to her strong personal faith. She went on to describe her experience the day before when she had been sent to the nuclear medicine department for a bone scan. She realized too late that she had not received her regularly scheduled injection of narcotics to relieve her pain before leaving the ward. During her half-day wait for the bone scan, she "prayed to God" to relieve her pain, and she said, "He did." The student-physician was silent as she talked about the effectiveness of her faith in helping her find jobs or relieving her pain. After the interview, he was asked what he thought about her comments on her religion. He looked blank and replied that he had not heard them. The instructor asked, "I wonder why you weren't able to hear them?" The student said, "I suppose it's because I don't believe in any of that crap."

Culture and Ethnicity

As we discussed in Chapter 4, patients from cultures other than that of the interviewer-clinician may behave in ways that are outside his or her usual experience. Although one should attempt to familiarize oneself with the practices and usual behavior in the health care situation of patients from other cultures, there is a danger in doing so. Racial and cultural stereotyping can lead the interviewer astray. While there are similarities in the behavior, attitudes, and practices of members of any culture or subculture, there are many individual exceptions. One should not expect a certain type of behavior from a given member of any ethnic or cultural group.

EMOTIONAL RESPONSES OF PATIENTS TO ILLNESS AND TO THE INTERVIEWER

Anxiety

Every illness produces a mixture of fear and anxiety in the patient. Some of the fears may be realistic, such as fear of pain, disability, death, or economic disaster if medical care is prolonged. Talking about such concerns to a sympathetic and supportive clinician usually will help reduce them to a manageable level. The difficulty is that many patients are hesitant to talk about their fears. This reticence tends to vary with the culture or subculture from which the patient comes. Patients who have been taught from earliest childhood to "be a man" or "be a good sport, don't complain" find it difficult to admit their fear. The necessity for a discreet inquiry about such fear is indicated when the patient does not express it directly but gives indirect evidence of concern. Since the term *fear* may be unacceptable, it is probably best to ask, "Are you worried about this?" Or, if the patient appears worried, though he has said nothing, it is usually preferable to confront him with a remark like, "You look worried." If the patient describes an event or symptom to which fear would be the usual response, but expresses none, a supportive inquiry may be helpful, something like, "That must have been frightening."

Anxiety, on the other hand, is usually considered to be a more diffuse feeling of apprehension that is difficult for the patient to attribute to a specific worry or fear. Fear and anxiety coexist in every illness and are normal or expectable responses. The most common sources of anxiety are feelings of helplessness, fear of dependency, an inability to accept warmth or tenderness, and fear of expressing anger.

Helplessness

The paradigm for the anxiety experienced by patients because they feel helpless is the situation of the surgical patient before an operation. No patient feels more helpless. The surgical patient knows that he will be immobilized, possibly unconscious, and during that period in which he can do nothing for himself and nothing to protect himself, a major "assault" will be made on his body. To some extent, every patient feels helpless. He is in the hands of someone, often not well-known to him, upon whom he must depend fully. Further, he cannot really make an objective assessment of the clinician's ability and knowledge. Even the relatively simple procedure of drawing blood or moving the patient from a hospital bed to a cart evokes some measure of anxiety because of helplessness. There are patients who can tolerate helplessness, who have basic trust in authorities and experts. There are other patients, however, whose self-esteem depends on being active, independent, and aggressive. To be helpless, to be confined to a bed, creates anxiety in such persons.

A patient's response to anxiety over helplessness usually is an intensification of his basic style of dealing with anxiety. A common reaction is to deny the anxiety and try to display just the opposite in one's actions. This response is designed to convince oneself and to communicate to others that one is not afraid. The idea that illness could result in being helpless is intolerable, and behavior designed to demonstrate the opposite is acted out. This is called *counterphobia*.

> A 42-year-old businessman succeeded in building a large diversified company largely through his own efforts. He was accustomed to being involved in a number of business deals at any given time and kept constantly in touch with all his operations, using his cellular phone heavily. When admitted to the hospital for examination, though seriously ill and in great discomfort, he was unable to lie in bed. He walked around the room, made business phone calls, and repeatedly interrupted the student who was attempting to conduct an initial diagnostic interview.

The usual indication that a patient is becoming very anxious is an intensification of his customary ways of coping with the world. For instance, the compulsive patient who has a need to be organized and to keep the world orderly and predictable will, on falling ill, probably become more compulsive and "fussy." He may insist on even more orderliness, predictability, neatness, or cleanliness than usual.

> A 22-year-old college student was admitted to the hospital for examination because of weakness, diarrhea, weight loss, abdominal pain, and evidence of anemia. He was a highly organized, orderly, and neat individual who was described as "compulsive." In the hospital, he complained of failure to collect his stool specimens and lack of punctuality with schedules, even though neither complaint was warranted. He became upset if he did not receive a new hospital gown each day, even though his was not dirty.

The anxious patient may be difficult to interview until the anxiety itself has been discussed. The patient who fears helplessness reacts best when the clinician's air of competence and concern indicates that he can be trusted; when he feels that he is receiving full and complete explanations in answer to his questions, reducing the ambiguity of the situation; and when efforts are made to reduce his sense of helplessness by allowing him to be as active as the situation permits.

Fear of Expressing Anger

There are many things that can provoke anger in a patient. A patient who arrives on time for a two o'clock appointment and then has a 45 minute wait in the reception room before the interview begins has a legitimate source of anger, for example. Anger can be an appropriate response to many of the circumstances of being a hospital patient. Inattentive personnel and failure to respond to the patient's needs are common, though not always intentional, occurrences in the hospital. But the situation of being helpless and dependent on others makes a patient especially sensitive to failure to meet his needs. Anger is a common response.

However, there are people who cannot permit themselves to express anger. With such a patient, anxiety over helplessness together with a fear of upsetting those on whom he must depend potentiates his fear of expressing anger and increases his anxiety. This is often reinforced by physicians and nurses whose behavior communicates to the patient that they will not accept his anger and may retaliate. The patient may even have had such experiences. Yet an important dimension of the clinician's role is to encourage expressions of such anger and to tolerate it even when it seems somewhat unreasonable. Only then can the patient's anxiety over his anger be reduced.

Depression

It is probable that depression accompanies every severe illness. Research on responses of children to separation from their mothers, on bereavement, and on psychosomatic illness all lend strong support to the view that depression is a psychophysiologic response to loss, including loss of self-esteem. Thus, while depression may be the underlying problem in a large proportion of those patients who consult their physician with complaints of fatigue, weakness, lack of energy, insomnia, backache, or headache, depression as a response to illness is equally common, if not more so.

Characteristically, depressed people have feelings of worthlessness, hopelessness, apathy, and guilt, together with a profoundly empty or lonely feeling. The depression will be manifested in the patient's manner, tone of voice, posture, and speech. Thinking is slow, speech is sparse, and voice volume is low. Hopelessness and sadness are reflected in the patient's drooping shoulders, downturned mouth, and lackluster eyes. A severely depressed patient will volunteer little and will respond to questions with brief, relatively uninformative answers. This will reduce the amount of information that can be obtained about the onset and development of the illness.

Many of these patients are people for whom having an illness is equivalent to being useless or "bad." Self-accusation may also be a component in depressive response to illness in instances where a patient believes he has not taken proper care of himself or has ignored advice given to him previously by his physician. Mild to moderate depression can be dealt with relatively easily during the interview, and good interviewing technique may bring some relief of the depressive symptoms. Severe depression can, however, be a major complication of the illness as well as of the interview itself.

Depressive reactions to illness may be characterized by apathetic withdrawal with silences. In such an instance a confrontation can be very helpful. A statement like, "You look very sad," or, "You look depressed," gives the patient the opportunity to talk about his depressed feelings. It is usually necessary to be more active in interviewing a depressed patient than one would be with other types of patients. More direct questions must be asked, and these are usually asked earlier in the interview than with a patient who is more communicative.

A special problem may be posed by the patient who begins to cry during an interview. Many clinicians find this uncomfortable. However, it may be of considerable help both to the patient and to the interviewer. Fighting tears often results in the patient's not being able to speak. Weeping, on the other hand, often afford relief of severe depressive feelings and may make it possible for the patient to resume his account. It may also help the patient to feel closer to the clinician. The appropriate response of the interviewer is to maintain a sympathetic silence while the patient cries and to respond with a supportive remark thereafter (e.g., "You must be feeling very bad"). A common error, usually stemming from the interviewer's discomfort, is to interrupt the crying with reassuring or supportive remarks before the patient has had a chance to "cry it out." It is better to wait patiently, to provide a tissue if necessary, to respond with sympathetic support after the patient has stopped crying, and to make no effort to resume the interview until then.

When a patient is on the verge of tears and this is clearly making it difficult for him to speak, it is often helpful to invite the crying with a confrontation: "You look like you are about to cry." The opportunity to cry, followed by the support offered by the clinician, will permit the interview to continue—and it can be therapeutic.

Denial

There are some patients whose customary way of dealing with frightening ideas or impulses is by never permitting them to enter their minds. On becoming ill, such patients must deny to themselves that such a thing has happened or that they need treatment. Consequently, they minimize or completely deny symptoms and consciously or unconsciously mislead the interviewer. Such patients are never completely aware of the degree to which they withhold, modify, or alter significant information. Other patients who are not ordinarily given to denial will consciously withhold or distort information because they are ashamed or fearful of the consequences of revealing it. A tendency to dismiss all symptoms with words such as "only" or "a little" should cue the interviewer to the possibility that the patient is using denial. Those patients who consciously withhold information often respond to some with evidence of discomfort or embarrassment, which reveals that a sensitive topic is under discussion about which the patient would rather not say too much.

Patients who tend to deal with unacceptable thoughts and feelings by denying them are not reliable informants about their own illnesses. If the interviewer clarifies his role at the outset and can create confidence in himself, he may be able to reduce the amount of denial used by the patient.

In subsequent interviews, with the development of a good clinician-patient relationship, the degree of denial used by the patient may be reduced markedly or, in the case of the conscious withholder, denial may disappear completely.

RESPONSES TO THE DOCTOR

The doctor-patient relationship tends to bring out attitudes and behavior reflecting previous relationships with other authorities or health care providers whose competence had an important bearing on the individual's comfort or welfare. This is also true of the nurse and the social worker. The more the patient feels that he is sick, and thus more helpless and dependent, the more likley it is that his attitude toward the doctor will reflect these previously formed attitudes. These attitudes are often manifested in ways that appear totally irrational to the interviewer. A patient who has had an angry, competitive relationship with his father, and who perceives the physician as a powerful authority, may become antagonistic, sarcastic, and competitive even though the doctor has done nothing that would ordinarily elicit such a response. Female clinicians often encounter irrational responses based on the patient's early experiences with being mothered or reflecting the patient's attitudes toward women. These can of course be positive or negative.

Because the patient is usually in pain, is anxious, and is aware of a threat, possibly of death or at least of impaired function, his need for attention and sympathy is far greater than it is at other times. He is therefore likely to respond in ways that reflect his relationship with his mother or other individuals to whom he turned for love and sympathy for his childhood discomforts. If these were satisfying experiences, he may be a relaxed and appropriately compliant patient. If they were frustrating experiences, he may approach the clinician with a mixture of fear, suspicion, and expectation of disappointment. If, as is so often the case with individuals who had chronic illness in childhood, the patient obtained attention and sympathy mostly through illness, he may embrace the role of patient and exploit it for as much sympathetic attention as he can get.

Still another determinant of the response to the clinician is the patient's past experience in getting health care. For some people, particularly those who obtained health care in clinics at large public hospitals, going to the doctor evokes memories of long waits, impersonal and dehumanizing encounters, and disregard for privacy. Memories of chronic illness in childhood that required painful procedures may make every visit to the doctor a dreaded event.

In other words, the interaction between the clinician and patient is highly charged with emotion. This will significantly affect the patient's interview behavior. Some of the more common responses that can pose problems for the interviewer include silence, excessive talkativeness, seductiveness, anger, aggressively demanding behavior, suspicion and distrust, and passive or dependent behavior.

The Silent Patient

With most patients, occasional silences are not uncommon during an interview. Silences of up to half a minute (which may feel quite protracted, even interminable, to the interviewer) usually mean that the patient is trying to recall something or is silently debating with himself whether to speak about a given topic or not. This is discussed at length in Chapter 2. Many interviewers, and most beginners, do not tolerate such silences well, and some interviewers never permit a patient the luxury of a period of silence. This may reflect, in part, the clinician's lack of comfort with the doctor-patient relationship since silences are not uncommon in conversations with people with whom one has a reasonably close social relationship. It may also partly reflect the clinician's feeling that he should perform his task—the interview—with maximum efficiency and dispatch. The most common reason clinicians interrupt silences is their own tension. Most interviewers tend to overestimate the duration of a silence. A useful exercise is to experiment with estimating the length of timed silences during interviews before actually checking the time. With practice one can learn to permit silence until the patient's tension suggests a confrontation or until the patient speaks.

The patient has been talking about her low back pain. The backache began during her first pregnancy, became worse after her second pregnancy, and is now constant. There is a note of marked discontent in her voice. After a few minutes she falls silent.

(*After about 20 seconds*)
INTERVIEWER: Anything else?
(*Silence for 20 seconds. The patient looks more depressed.*)
INTERVIEWER: You look quite unhappy.
(*Silence for 15 seconds*)
PATIENT: I feel just awful. The children are just too much for me. All that lifting and carrying hurts my back so much. I get no help from Jack. (*Tears appear.*) Oh, I just knew if I talked about it, I'd start to cry.

There are patients, however, who remain silent for long periods of time, or fall silent frequently. The interviewer may have the feeling that he is constantly pushing the patient to keep communication going. This usually means that the patient is seriously depressed, which may be part of the illness or a response to it. Questioning about symptoms of depression, as well as careful observation for the classic signs of depression in the patient's facial expression, posture, and attitude, will clarify the diagnosis. Prolonged and repeated silences may also be a manifestation of an organic brain disease or a psychosis.

There are instances when prolonged or repeated silences result from poor interviewing technique. Clumsy or insensitive handling of the opening phase of the interview, too many specific questions asked too early in the interview, too many interruptions, or tactless remarks may result in silences and brief answers, which reflect withdrawal and an offended patient.

The Excessively Talkative Patient

A most difficult problem for both the beginner and the experienced interviewer is the excessively talkative patient. This patient may be seen as a barrier to getting a day's work done with reasonable efficiency. He very often frustrates the clinician's efforts to get sufficient relevant information within reasonable time limits, and usually irritates the inter-

KENT
TEMPLEMAN
LIBRARY

viewer. Such a patient slows down the clinician and imposes a burden of self-restraint upon him. This is not, however, the only reason that such patients are irritating to the interviewer. There is usually an aggressive quality to such a patient's communication, which has a controlling or dominating effect. One type of excessively talkative patient is the obsessional individual who insists on giving an overly detailed account, omitting nothing, not even the most trivial detail. In interviewing such a patient, one must be careful to avoid overfacilitating through encouraging nods, gestures, and phrases. Relatively specific questions should be introduced earlier in the sequence of the interview than might be done with a less obsessive patient. The interviewer should limit his show of interest when the patient is supplying a great deal of trivial detail but show greater interest where appropriate. Courteous interruptions when enough information has been obtained about a given point, followed by another question, will also keep the interview focused and make it possible to accomplish the interviewing task within a reasonable period of time.

There are patients, however, who will not be hurried. Their obsessive need to recall detail and to present all of it to the interviewer is so great that attempts to focus the interview fail to hasten the patient's account to any measurable degree. Impatience or anger on the part of the interviewer will only complicate the relationship and make matters worse. In such cases, it is best to relax and to accept the situation as gracefully as possible.

The patient, an obsessive 42-year-old man, was describing the pressure of each job he had after leaving a somewhat subordinate position in a large industry for a series of executive positions with small, federally funded community projects. Midway through each such description it became apparent that the pressures were similar and the patient's symptoms were identical each time they recurred. In describing the third recurrence, the interviewer decided to interrupt.

PATIENT: And then the stomach pains began again. First I began to notice that I'd get nauseated after breakfast . . .
INTERVIEWER: (*Interrupting*) Were the symptoms the same as the first two times?
PATIENT: Oh, yes. (*Goes on to recount them all, once again.*)

The interviewer took a deep breath, settled back, and, glancing at his watch began to rearrange mentally the remainder of his day.

Another type of excessive talkativeness is encountered in the patient who rambles. Often elderly, or simply garrulous, this patient does not behave as an obsessive patient does, but he seems to be poorly organized. With this type of patient, one should interrupt when the patient wanders away from the topic at hand unless the patient is in fact supplying information that appears indirectly relevant. It may be necessary to refocus the patient's attention frequently. There is still another type of very talkative patient whose chattering quality betrays his underlying anxiety. A friendly, reassuring, or supportive comment about the patient's evident anxiety is often sufficient to reduce it.

Since for many people verbal communication is a way of controlling and reducing the freedom of the other individual, there is danger with some patients that the interview can become a battle of wills. To get the job done, and to reassure the patient that the interviewer is, in fact, capable of carrying out diagnosis and treatment, the interviewer should not allow control of the interview to slip into the patient's hands. On the other hand, an interview should be conducted sensitively enough that the patient does not feel dominated or overcontrolled. Most patients respect a clinician whose manner suggests strength and self-assurance. But there are individuals who cannot stand the feeling of being subservient. This, in itself, need not pose a problem. But when such a patient cannot accept a relationship of mutual participation, the relationship can be a severe trial of patience for the clinician.

Not all excessive talkativeness represents an attempt to dominate the other person. Some patients feel a kind of closeness when talking. They tend to be lonely individuals who cannot tolerate silence and who feel that there is a bond between them and the clinician if someone is speaking. This is detectable by the interviewer, who will feel it as a "sticky," clinging kind of communication. Bed-ridden patients suffering from chronic disease will often make every effort to prolong interviews and keep talking, fearing that the interviewer will go away.

The excessively talkative patient poses a particularly difficult problem in the managed care setting. Time constraints may require that the doctor become very active in limiting the length of the patient's answers.

The Paranoid Patient

Occasionally, the clinician will encounter a patient who has a paranoid personality. Such individuals are chronically angry, suspicious, and distrustful, and they easily become convinced that some person or agency has a malign plan or design directed against them. They tend to brood, become depressed over real and fancied injustices, carry grudges, ruminate about wrongs experienced years before, and quickly assume that the clinician's intention cannot be trusted. Such patients may or may not be delusional, but in either case they are most difficult to interview. Any topic that arouses their suspicion or provokes angry accusations should not be pursued. Warm and reassuring behavior tends to be threatening to these patients and provokes more paranoia. It is best to maintain a friendly but cool and detached neutrality with paranoid patients. Tactful firmness, avoidance of angry responses to the patient, and consistency help to build whatever sense of trust the patient may be capable of feeling. Reassurance and support, on the other hand, which might be warmly received by most patients, is usually very upsetting to the paranoid patient.

A Note on Evasive, Indirect and Embarrassed Patients

Sensitivity to the patient's experience in the interview dictates that one may not always proceed at once to the task of gathering data about the patient's present complaints and problems. When a patient shows evidence of evasiveness or indirectness, there is a natural tendency to push harder for information, to make one's questions more specific and more pointed, or to press for more precise and detailed descriptions. This is a mistake. There is usually some topic or concern that the patient must get out of the way first. Evasiveness or indirectness frequently means that the patient is ambivalent about talking about something, knowing that it would probably be helpful but fearing to speak openly. The patient may be embarrassed, feel guilty, or fear that something about to be revealed will not be kept in confidence. The skilled interviewer will, at this point, abandon the direct inquiry and shift to a discussion of the patient's behavior and apparent discomfort. A comment like, "You seem to be having a great deal of difficulty talking about this," will often open a discussion of the source of the difficulty. After the discussion it should be possible to continue the inquiry with less reticence on the patient's part. Other patients have difficulty talking to anyone and will require more direct questioning and specific inquiries to elicit details than the usual patient.

The patient who states early in the interview that he'll be happy to answer the doctor's questions may appear to the inexperienced interviewer to be especially cooperative when actually he is frequently hoping to avoid certain areas of information. His is not a cooperative attitude. He is saying, in effect, "I won't volunteer a thing." Similarly, other patients, basically passive or dependent individuals, have great difficulty volunteering anything and prefer to be led, to be asked questions to which they will supply answers rather than to volunteer information. This is often experienced by the interviewer as demanding behavior, which is exactly what it is. If the clinician relationship continues, these patients are likely to become more and more openly demanding. It is important for the clinician to understand the reason for the demand and to maintain an appropriate distance. In this way he will be able to avoid becoming angry and possibly punitive.

CLINICIAN'S BEHAVIOR AND PATIENT'S RESPONSE

As we have already noted, patients all have a certain amount of anxiety and often depression. There are ways to reduce the discomfort of the patient. These include the clearly indicated interest of the clinician, a friendly and supportive demeanor, an open-ended style of interviewing, and facilitating expression of the patient's feelings.

Certain other types of clinician behavior can have the opposite effect, that of increasing the patient's anxiety, apprehension, and depression. These include being aloof, looking at the clinical folder or bedside chart rather than the patient, treating the patient with disrespect, being abrupt, and failing to respond with support when a patient has expressed strong emotion, such as unhappiness or fearfulness.

In summary, the clinician's emotional response to the patient's behavior can be positive or negative, but it is never neutral. In every case the clinician must try to be aware of it, recognize it as a possible hazard to an effective clinician-patient relationship if ignored, and maintain awareness of his or her role as physician. The patient's behavior is part of the data that is being gathered.

6

INTERVIEWING CHILDREN

Karen Brummel-Smith, M.D.

KEY POINTS

1. Talk to children directly, using warm-up questions and non-threatening touch.
2. Tailor interviewing techniques and question complexity to the child's age.
3. Identify the parent's "main worry" through open-ended questions.
4. Use patience in desensitizing the frightened child; use play, reassurance, and multiple visits if necessary.
5. Assure confidentiality to adolescents; discuss home, education, activities, drugs, sex, and suicide risk (HEADSS technique).

Perhaps nowhere in the practive of medicine is the physician required to be more flexible than in the care of children. When interviewing pediatric patients and their families, doctors must be prepared for the varied expectations that young patients bring to the medical encounter. Children may enter the doctor-patient relationship with fears and fantasies about what will be "done to them" during a visit to the doctor. The physician must get onto the child's level, both figuratively and often physically if trust with that patient is to be established. In addition, virtually every visit by a child requires addressing not only the child's needs, but also the accompanying parent's. As children grow older, their questions and concerns may diverge more from those of the parent. This chapter examines these unique aspects of the pediatric interview and provides information about how the doctor can successfully manage the needs and expectations of both children and their parents. Special attention is paid to interviewing the unusually shy or frightened child, assessing the abused child, and interviewing the adolescent patient.

WHAT IS DIFFERENT ABOUT INTERVIEWING CHILDREN?

Setting the Stage

Though the pediatric visit parallels in many ways a visit with an older patient, there are many significant differences in conducting the pediatric interview. Unlike adults, most children require a warm-up period in which they can become familiar with the physician and the office setting. If available, a special pediatric exam room is helpful for interviewing and examining young children. Appropriate decor might include bright colors, pictures of familiar children's characters, or a small variety of toys. Some children may feel uncomfortable with the formality of the doctor's white coat. At the physician's discretion it may be left off for the pediatric visit.

Putting the Patient at Ease

The physician should make every effort to "get on the child's level" by sitting or crouching down next to the patient and addressing him or her by name. The opening segment of the interview should be approached in an unhurried fashion, delaying focus on the medical aspects of the visit. A "warm-up cluster" of questions may be asked to help set the child at ease.[1] This can include inquiring about school, siblings, favorite games, or toys. If a child has brought a toy from home, asking about it is an excellent way to begin to get to know the child. Even an infant can be greeted in a soothing tone of voice and spoken to by name with direct eye contact. This will be helpful in setting the child at ease and will reassure the parent about your concern for his or her child.

Nonthreatening touch at this stage of the visit is also helpful, but avoid the stereotypic pat on the head. Tickling should be used cautiously as it can be frightening and annoying to children. Look instead for genuine ways to approach the child physically, touching his arm to look at a wristwatch, reaching for her feet to comment on her Minnie Mouse shoes.

In the initial moments of the physician's interaction with the family, it is important to observe the nonverbal communication among family members. If several are present, are there obvious alliances between family members? Who sits with whom? How is the patient regarded within the group? Is the prevailing feeling in the room relaxed, tense, somber? Does the child (or children) appear particularly frightened or withdrawn? These observations can be clues to the family's dynamics and/or style of coping with illness.

Addressing the Child

Perhaps the most common error in interviewing children is failure to address the child directly. This not only limits important information that will be supplied by the child, but also shifts the physician's attention away from focused observation of him or her. Many physicians may feel more comfortable in conventional discourse with the parent and may be impatient with the sometimes more circuitous style required when interacting with a child. The physician may feel uncertain about what level of questioning is appropriate for a child of a given age.

A basic understanding of stages of childhood development can be helpful in allaying these concerns (Table 6.1). While first words are usually spoken around one year of age, typically more is comprehended by a child of this age. Speaking to a one-year-old in simple phrases is appropriate, despite the fact that he cannot yet respond verbally. By the age of 24 months, the average child is speaking in two- or three-word phrases and has a vocabulary of about 270 words. Preschoolers' expanding vocabulary allows them to speak in concrete terms about the "here and now," but their concept of time and understanding of past tense is

TABLE 6.1. Development of Children's Communication Skills

Age	Language Skills
1 Year	Can be spoken to in simple phrases, does not respond verbally
2 Years	Vocabulary of 200–300 words, can respond in simple phrases
3–4 Years	Responds in full sentences, understands "who," "what," and "where" questions, poor conceptualization of past tense and past events
5–6 Years	Good grasp of past tense, can recall and report events, understands "when," "why," and "how"

limited. Questions about chronology of symptoms or use of complex past tense verbs will be confusing for the preschooler. By age six, most children are able to communicate effectively about past events. A good rule of thumb is that a child can comprehend "where, what, and who" questions by age three, but cannot consistently respond to "why, when, or how" until the age of five or six.[2]

Careful word choice on the part of the physician is extremely important in the pediatric visit. Complex sentence structure and medical jargon should be avoided. If a young child is asked about nausea, vomiting, and abdominal pain, he will likely stare blankly back at the physician. It can be helpful to listen for clues in the child's or parent's speech as to how the child refers to body parts. (Mother: "Tell the doctor about your bellyache, Joey.") If such clues are absent, use colloquial rather than medical terms, asking simple, concrete questions like, "Does your belly hurt now? Did you throw up at home?"

Physicians may not realize that words used commonly in medical settings are unfamiliar to many lay people. In a large study of pediatric emergency room visits, it was found that simple medical terms were often inadequately explained, leading to confusion of the parents. When a mother was told that her son had to be "admitted for a workup," she was unaware that her child needed stay in the hospital and unsure about the plan for treatment. The physician must use terms that will be understood. "Electrolytes," "cardiologist," "parasitic infections," and "lumbar punctures" will likely be perceived as a foreign language both by children and by all but the most educated parents. [3]

Tailoring Interview Techniques to the Younger Patient

Standard interviewing techniques can be effectively utilized in the pediatric interview. Some must be tailored to the age of the child. Empathy and attentive listening are appropriate in all encounters. ("I understand you're feeling kind of scared about having your tonsils out, Alex.") Confrontation is unlikely to be of benefit in talking with a young child. It can be a valuable tool in working with adolescent patients, but should be reserved until a sense of relationship with the physician has been established. Therapeutic silence in the course of an interview is unlikely to be of use in talking with a child, particularly an adolescent. Reflective statements may be helpful in encouraging a child of school age or older to further clarify the information given. (Colleen, age twelve: "I hate wearing this cast to school, it really bugs me!" Doctor: "So that cast is really bugging you.") Summarizing statements can be particularly reassuring to the adolescent and will communicate that the physician is paying careful attention to the patient's concerns. ("I want to make sure I'm understanding you, Carlos. The things that bother you most are having no privacy at home, and wondering if it's safe to have sex with your girlfriend.")

Open-ended questions are important in interviewing children. Too often the physician underestimates the ability of the child to generate his own answers and will resort to yes-or-no questions. As with adult patients, the physician's style of questioning can bias and limit a child's response. It is not uncommon for somatic symptoms in a child to represent deeper underlying emotional, social, or family problems. [4,5] Questions like, "Are you coughing at night?" or, "Does your throat hurt when you swallow?" may be important for understanding the biological dimension of the illness, but they are unlikely to uncover hidden information about the etiology or exacerbation of an illness.

DOCTOR: Your mom says you've been feeling sick. Can you tell me about
it?

ARTHUR, age eight: I've been coughin' for two weeks, but all she cares
about is that stupid new boyfriend of hers.

Special Circumstances

Children's language is best understood in the context of their age, development, and familiar activities. Younger children's speech and thought
patterns in particular differ from those of adults. Prepositions, explanations, and logical progression of ideas may be absent from children's
responses. Becky, age four, is being seen in the office for evaluation of
headaches.

DOCTOR: What makes your head feel better, Becky?
BECKY: When I drink special juice and the clowns sing Zip-e-Doo and
dance up in the sky.

Becky's response could be viewed as confabulation without further
inquiry. Upon talking further with Becky's mother, the physician
learned that Becky has a musical mobile that hangs above her bed and
plays a soothing melody. Her mother gives her liquid acetaminophen
mixed in juice, and Becky lies in bed listening to her favorite song.

The unusually shy or frightened child presents a unique challenge to
a physician seeing him or her for the first time. Children may have had a
number of previous experiences with medical care. A past hospitalization, a painful procedure, or simply the memory of a gruff doctor may
color a child's willingness to engage in a relationship with a new physician. The manifestations of the child's fear may range from quiet reser-
vation to screaming wildly at the sight of any health care provider.
Patience and creativity on the clinician's part are essential in these situations. If the child is extremely uncomfortable, the physician must re-
define the agenda for the visit and treat the fear as if it were any other
problem for which care is required. If necessary, all other expectations
for the visit should be abandoned (unless, of course, the child is acutely
ill) and attention directed at setting the child at ease. Any promises made

to the child toward this end, (i.e., "Let's just talk today, Ethan," or, "I promise we won't give you any shots today") must be scrupulously kept. Nothing will be gained, and further harm will probably be done, if the physician simply tries to push through the child's resistance. The physician should be realistic in attempting to establish a relationship with a fearful child. An explanation can be given to the parents that it may take several visits before the child begins to feel more confortable. Scheduling one or two visits to desensitize the child to the medical environment may be valuable. It may be tempting for the physician to retreat into talking solely with the parents when confronted with a shy or frightened child. While this may ultimately be necessary, it should not be done prematurely. Any success, however small, in interacting with the child will likely serve to diminish the problem on subsequent visits.

An attempt should be made to ascertain the reasons that the child is fearful. Both the parent and child may be questioned about this. Verbal reassurance should be given to the child in a positive framework. ("I'd like to play with you for a few minutes today, David," rather than, "I'm not going to hurt you.") Physical touch should be avoided until the child shows signs of increased comfort with the physician. In this setting, it may be helpful to have a doll with which the child can show how he or she feels. The physician can use the doll in the initial interview to ask both emotional and physical questions of the child. ("Do you think the doll feels scared, too? Does this doll's tummy hurt?")

INTERVIEWING PARENTS

Discussing Psychosocial Concerns

Parents arrive with many agendas when they bring their children to the doctor's office. To make the visit successful, it is the interviewer's job to identify the concerns and expectations of the parent. Even though the present complaint may be a physical problem, in many cases it is accompanied by deeper psychosocial, developmental, or behavioral concerns. A large body of research has shown that parental satisfaction with the pediatric care their child has received is markedly enhanced by the willingness of the physician to discuss the parents' psychosocial concerns about their child.[3,6,7] One study indicated that in seventy percent of mothers who brought their child to a pediatrician's office, the primary concern was psychosocial, ranging from personality development, discipline, mother-child interactions, adjustment to divorce and other life changes, to transition to adolescence. Three-fourths of the mothers in this study failed to raise these concerns with their doctor. When questioned about this, they cited a variety of reasons. They did not know their doctor could help or felt he was too busy, not qualified, or unwilling to help. Some denied needing help or said they were too embarrassed to discuss their worries with their physician. For those who did voice their concerns, the physician's expression of interest was the most important determinant of communication.[8]

This study and others reveal how the behavior of the physician influences the content of the interview. Often physicians convey subtle or overt preferences for dealing with problems that are strictly physical.[8,9] A frequent mistake is to assume that the first problem raised in the interview is the most important one. Often the first issue discussed in the interview will be a physical symptom or concern about biological disease, as parents have been socialized to think that these are appropriate problems to be addressed in the pediatrician's office. If the parent or child later spontaneously expresses a psychosocial concern, he or she may be interrupted by the physician and steered back to the physical realm. Such premature termination of this vein of discussion will inhibit the patient's subsequently broaching such topics.[10] If the initial complaint is taken at face value and followed with direct questioning about it, the true reason for the visit may never be elucidated.

Mrs. Lorens has come to her family doctor concerned about her colicky two-month-old baby.

MRS. LORENS: Doctor, I don't know what to do about Elizabeth's spitting up. It seems like she does it all the time. And she cries so much. Sometimes I just want to scream at her, but she's just a baby and I know it isn't her fault. Do you think something's wrong with my breast milk? Could it be hurting her somehow?

DOCTOR: How much is she spitting up? Is it every feeding?

MRS. LORENS: Well, I guess it's not every time. It seems like a lot, though. It just seems like she's so tense. Her tummy gets real tight and she turns all red and sometimes she just screams for hours. I just wonder if my breast milk is bad.

DOCTOR: It sounds like Elizabeth has a classic case of colic. Most babies will outgrow it by the time they're three months old. I don't think it's your breast milk, but you can make sure to avoid spicy foods that might aggravate her.

Here the doctor has provided Mrs. Lorens with some valuable information and anticipatory guidance, but has focused the interaction solely in the biological realm. He could have responded in a more open-ended fashion to facilitate Mrs. Lorens' expression of deeper concerns.

DOCTOR: It sounds as if you're pretty worried about Elizabeth.

MRS. LORENS: Oh . . . (*teary and appearing embarrassed*) . . . it's just so hard with her. Sometimes I just don't know what to do. My neighbor told me about her two-month-old niece who died from that Sudden Infant Death thing. Some nights I just can't sleep worrying if she's gonna stop breathing. My husband says I'm a basket case. Maybe he was right. Maybe we should never have had her in the first place.

DOCTOR: Mrs. Lorens, it sounds as if you and your husband are feeling a lot of stress with the new baby. It's very common for families to go through this, and to wonder if there might be something that they are doing that is making it worse. I think it's important for us to spend more time talking about these things than we can spend today. Perhaps you and your husband might consider coming in together to talk about how things are going.

With supportive confrontation the physician has elicited the range of problems that Mrs. Lorens is experiencing with her new baby. The stress on her marriage, her self-doubts as a new mother, and her feelings of worry about and anger toward her child can be explored further in this or subsequent visits. At this point the physician can offer guidance about colic and breastfeeding and provide information about Sudden Infant Death Syndrome. In this scenario, Mrs. Lorens is much more likely to leave the doctor's office with the feeling that her doctor is genuinely concerned about her life and her family.

Korsch suggests that one of the most important tasks of the physician in the pediatric interview is to identify the parent's "main worry."[3] In her study the two most valuable questions used to uncover this information were, "What has worried you most about your child's illness?" and, "Why did that worry you?" Commonly parents are worried that for some reason they are to blame for their child's problem. It behooves the physician to explore these issues with the parent (as with Mrs. Lorens) and to provide reassurance and relief from self-blame whenever appropriate. It may take very little probing to reveal the parent's deepest concerns when the physician manifests genuine concern and interviews in an open-ended way.

The inexperienced physician may feel overwhelmed by the myriad of issues raised by such a parent in response to open-ended questions. It is important to remember that not all problems raised have to (or can) be resolved in one or even several visits. Simply the doctor's acknowledgment of the scope of the parent's concerns can be therapeutic.

A common misconception is that allowing parents to share their psychosocial concerns will take too much time. Beckman and Frankel found that most physician interruptions of patients' complaints took place between 5 to 50 seconds following the physician's initial request for information.[10] When patients were allowed to freely elaborate their concerns in response to an open-ended question, completed responses took no longer than two and one-half minutes.

Understanding Diverse Families

It is important in talking with a parent to avoid making assumptions about who constitutes that patient's family. As discussed in the chapter on interviewing families, there are many types of groups that patients may define as their family.

> Leanne Porter, a first-time mother, has newly relocated. She brings her three-year-old, Josh, to the pediatrician for a well-child check-up.

DOCTOR: Good morning, Mrs. Porter. I'm Dr. Mary Singleton.

LEANNE: Good morning. Actually, doctor, you could just call me Leanne. I'm not married.

DOCTOR: Oh, I see. I'm sorry for the mistake.

(Later in the interview)

DOCTOR: I'll need to get some family history about your son. Can you tell me about your health history and the child's father's history?

LEANNE: Well, his father is . . . uh . . . not really involved. I don't know anything about his history.

DOCTOR: Well, it must be a challenge for you raising a rambunctious three-year-old as a single parent.

LEANNE: Yes it is.

Here the doctor has tried to be empathetic, but has failed to learn anything about Josh and Leanne's family.

DOCTOR: Good morning. It's nice to meet you. Hello Josh. I'm Dr. Mary Singleton.

(Later in the interview)

DOCTOR: I'd like to learn a little bit more about both of you and your family. Can you tell me who lives at home?

LEANNE: Well, *(appearing a little uncomfortable)*, there's Josh and me and my friend Linda.

DOCTOR: Your friend, Linda?

LEANNE: Uh, yes. we've been roommates for the last seven years.

DOCTOR: I've found that many of my patients with same-sex roommates are gay or lesbian. I'm wondering if this applies to you?

LEANNE: Well, yes it does. Linda is my lover and Josh thinks of her as his mom, too. They're so great together! *(Smiling and appearing more relaxed.)* But my parents, unfortunately, want nothing to do with us. It makes me so sad that Josh can't just have a normal relationship with his grandparents.

In the first scenario, the physician's false assumption has likely inhibited Leanne from sharing her sexual orientation. It will be difficult for Dr. Singleton to provide comprehensive care for Josh without knowing about the family in which he lives. With the increasing frequency of

divorce, blended families, and shared custody of children, it is impera-
tive that the physician ask questions in a nonjudgmental way. It is also
valuable to ascertain if there are other significant people in the child's
life—a day-care provider, a neighbor, or a teacher who is close to the
child. A family genogram (see Fig. 3.1) may be helpful when living
arrangements and relationships are complex.[11]

PAST MEDICAL HISTORY

The past medical history is an important part of the initial pediatric
interview (Table 6.2). The physician should review the prenatal and
birth history as well as significant illnesses of the child and the parents.
Illnesses during pregnancy, the circumstances and complications of the
birth, and the mother's feeling about the pregnancy should be reviewed.
Pertinent childhood diseases, history of surgery, and immunization status, including beliefs and values about immunization, should be discussed. It is important to ask about any behavioral problems. With
school-aged children, the physician should inquire about school performance and adjustment to the educational environment.

A host of environmental factors may put the child at risk; thus, the
physician should ask about smoking and alcohol use in the home, risk of
lead poisoning (particularly in homes built before the 1940s when
leaded paints were used), and potential exposure to gasoline, solvents, or
firearms. Parents should be advised about the risks of accidental poisoning, particularly with younger children. This is a good time in the
interchange to ask about the use of automobile seat belts and car seats for

TABLE 6.2. Components of a Pediatric Medical History

Parent's illness	Immunizations
Prenatal history	History of accidents
Birth history	Environmental exposures
Childhood illnesses	Safety issues
Surgeries	Discipline style
Behavior problems	Education history

the younger child. A history of frequent accidents is significant in any child and is correlated with high levels of family stress. [12] The physician should inquire about the parents' beliefs and practices regarding discipline, making note of any elements of the history that may suggest that a child is or has been abused. It may be helpful to ask the parents what they enjoy most about their child and, conversely, what troubles them most.

Finally, always assume that the parent has questions. And remember that the child may have questions as well. "What questions do you have?" gives more permission to raise concerns than the typical, "Do you have any questions?" It is important to pay attention to questions asked by the parent that the physician feels may already have been adequately answered. A repeated question is a clear indication that the physician has not effectively explained the answer. The information should be communicated again, if possible by using simpler language or by illustrating the point with an example or by drawing a picture. Simply repeating the answer in the same way it was explained before may produce the same confusion in the parent. At the end of the interview it is valuable to add, "Is there anything important I should know about your child or your family that we haven't yet discussed?"

INTERVIEWING ADOLESCENTS

There is perhaps no more turbulent time in the human life cycle than adolescence. The tasks of individuating from parents, coping with peer pressure, and adapting to a changing body made this a period of both confusion and enormous excitement. The risks that adolescents face in the 1990s exceed those of the generations before them, including those experienced by most physicians in their own youth. Therefore, the physician caring for adolescents should keep in mind the unique challenges that young people face today. There may be no better education in these issues than frank talk with adolescents themselves.

Adolescence is a time of growth and development, increased risk-taking, and considerable emotional upheaval, but it is not characterized by a large number of physical ailments. Nonetheless, teenagers are unlikely to come to the doctor's office with complaints like, "I'm smoking too much pot," or, "I'm feeling so depressed since my parents split up, I don't know if I can go on." Physical symptoms or problems like viral infections, sexually transmitted disease, injuries, or the need for birth control usually bring adolescents through the office door. It is the physician's job to make sure that the evaluation of the adolescent doesn't end there.

Confidentiality

The cornerstone of the interview with the adolescent is confidentiality. Young people need to know that their deepest concerns will be held in confidence. If a doctor is to become privy to the risks, emotions, and behaviors that might impinge upon an adolescent's health, the teenager must feel confident that the information will go no further. It must be stated very clearly to the adolescent that all matters, with the exception of physical or sexual abuse, and suicidal or homicidal behavior or intent, will be kept in strict confidence. This raises a dilemma for the interviewer of the adolescent who comes in for evaluation with a parent. While in general it is recommended that family members first be interviewed together, this may severely hinder the adolescent's willingness to speak frankly to the physician. Another strategy is to exclude family members, including parents, from the interview unless permission is given by the adolescent. This communicates clearly to the patient from the onset that the physician identifies the adolescent and her perception of her own problems as the primary reason for the visit. While many teenagers will give their permission for a parent or others to participate in the interview, they should always be interviewed privately for at least part of the discussion. Because of the progressively decreasing age of onset of risk-taking behaviors (drug and alcohol use, smoking, sexual exploration), the clinician should consider a private segment of the interview for any child over the age of ten. Beyond the age of twelve, the patient must be given the opportunity to speak frankly with the physician about his or her concerns. It is important to note that many adolescents will not necessarily speak in a forthcoming way to the physician about their deepest concerns on an initial visit. But the fact that the doctor

makes the opportunity available increases the likelihood of greater dis-
closure on subsequent visits.

The HEADSS Interview

An excellent technique for organizing the psychosocial interview with
an adolescent has the acronym HEADSS (Table 6.3). Designed by
Berman and further developed by Goldenring and Cohen, this six-step
acronym focuses on evaluation of the *H*ome environment, *E*ducation
and employment, peer *A*ctivities, *D*rugs, *S*exuality, and *S*uicide/
depression. Many of the following questions that explore these areas
were suggested by Goldenring and Cohen. [13]

In each of these segments of the adolescent interview, a more
physician-centered approach is necessary. Simple open-ended questions
may not stimulate young patients to be thorough in their responses. For
example, "Tell me about your home," is likely to yield the response,
"Oh, it's O.K." It is important to be relatively specific with the adolescent. "Who lives with you?" "Where?" "Do you have your own room?"
"Have you moved recently or frequently?" "What are your relationships
like at home?" Try to ascertain if the adolescent has someone at home to
trust and talk to. It is important not to make assumptions about the
nature of a young person's home life. Ask about history of running away,
living on the streets, or institutionalization.

"How are you doing in school?" is a common question posed to
young people in the course of an interview. Again, this question is likely
to be answered, "O.K." Better choices are asking what the teenager does

TABLE 6.3. The HEADSS Psychosocial
Interview for Adolescents

H	home environment
E	education, employment
A	activities
D	drugs
S	sexuality
S	suicide, depression

well in school, what is hard for him or her. Asking for specific grades gives a more objective view of the adolescent's struggles and strengths in school. Inquiring about a recent change in grades is important as suddenly worsening grades may be associated with depression, increased suicide risk, and/or substance abuse. In middle and late adolescence many teenagers will already have had summer jobs or have begun to think about future employment. Similar questions about strengths and weaknesses and relationships at work are appropriate.

The young person's activities can be explored by asking simple questions like, "What do you and your friends like to do together?" or, "How do you spend your free time?" Again, details of the patient's activities are important. A girl who is vague about her activities away from home and school may be masking the fact that she does not have friends and is depressed.

The manner of initiating a discussion about behaviors such as drug and alcohol use and sexual relationships is extremely important. A nonjudgmental tone is obligatory to obtain any information. A format for presenting these questions that gives the adolescent greater permission to respond honestly is to frame the question in light of the behaviors of their peers. For example: "Many young people your age experiment with drugs, alcohol, or cigarettes. Have you or your friends ever tried them?" If the answer is yes, ask, "What have you tried?" Given the risk for contracting the HIV virus through intravenous drug use, it is important to ask, "Have you ever used a needle to get high?" In broaching the subject of sexuality, one might ask, "Most young people become interested in sexual relationships at about your age. Have you had any experiences with boys, girls, or both?" or, "Since sexual activity can affect your health, I am interested in learning as much about you as I can. Can you tell me about your sex life?" Patients of both sexes should be asked whether they have been touched sexually in unwelcomed or uncomfortable ways.

The physician seeing adolescent patients must assume that the patients are at risk for sexually transmitted disease, including HIV infection. With a sexually active teenager, ask specifically about use of condoms. Regardless of whether or not an adolescent reports being sexually active, information about safe sex, birth control, and abstinence can be offered.

The physician should have a high index of suspicion for depression in adolescents. Altered presentation of depression is common in young people. Symptoms like worsening school performance, truancy, substance abuse, severe family problems, and sudden change in circle of friends should be viewed as potential indicators of depression. Adolescents struggling with depression are at risk for suicide and are unlikely to volunteer thoughts or plans to harm themselves. In this case, it is important to ask directly about suicidal thoughts. "Have you ever felt so down that you've thought about killing yourself?" Specifics about a plan, previous attempts, and access to the means of carrying out a potential plan should be assessed.

Eating Disorders

Finally, the physician interviewing adolescent girls should have a high index of suspicion of the presence of eating disorders. Anorexia nervosa, characterized by a compulsive pursuit of thinness and a distorted body image, may have a prevalence as high as 1 in 200 adolescent girls, particularly middle-to-upper-class Caucasians.[14] Bulimia, a related disorder of binge eating and subsequent purging through vomiting, may be seen by itself or in association with anorexia. The abuse of laxatives to control weight may be associated with both syndromes. Though not classically anorexic or bulimic, many girls are excessively preoccupied with weight loss and can benefit from discussing issues of body image with their physician. While anorexic patients in the later stages of the disease are more visible because of their marked weight loss, teenagers in the early stages cannot be identified by their appearance. Most bulimics are of normal weight and will only be identified through careful interviewing.

Referring to an adolescent's peer group is a good way to explore this subject. "Some girls your age are very worried about their weight. Have you been concerned about this yourself?" "Some girls your age force themselves to vomit or use laxatives to keep their weight down. Do you have friends who have tried that? Have you ever tried it?" Eating disorders are commonly associated with depression; anorexia, in particular, is associated with isolation from family and excessive anxiety about achievement. The interview should explore these areas, as well as suicidal impulses.

IDENTIFYING CHILD ABUSE

While a thorough review of the evaluation of children for suspected child abuse lies beyond the scope of this chapter, some basic approaches will be presented here. In many cases primary care physicians are the first to identify the risks for, or presence of, abuse in their patients. It can take the form of neglect or physical, emotional, or sexual abuse.

Careful observation of children in relation to their parents is often revealing. Does the child seem visibly frightened of any family member? Does he or she appear excessively sad or display an absence of emotion when one would expect to see an emotional response (i.e., no response to a painful procedure)? In the interview does the child have more difficulty than expected by age in responding to questions about a suspicious symptom? Does the child give repetitive "No" responses that may represent denial rather than simple answers about what happened?

Physicians must decide how to proceed with an interview when they suspect that the parents who have brought their child in may be responsible for abusing that child. Direct accusations should be avoided since they will commonly cause parents to become defensive. One approach is to raise the question in general terms. "Mr. and Mrs. Jones, I have some concerns about Julia. This is not the kind of injury that usually occurs accidentally. Is it possible someone may have hurt her?" The parents' nonverbal communication in response to this type of question may be as important as the content of their answer. Do the parents respond hesitantly? Are there discrepancies between two parents' tone of response or explanation of the injury? Is the explanation consistent with the injury? If both parents are present, does one answer all the questions? If a physician has a high degree of suspicion that the parent is responsible for the abuse and may pressure the child to be silent (or abuse the child further) if pressed to discuss it, the physician may choose to withhold his or her suspicion from the parents. This would be appropriate only in the case of mild injuries. Here the doctor might say, "Your son appears to have some worries. I think he could be helped by counseling. I'd like to arrange for him to talk with someone in more detail about them."[15]

Not all suspicious injuries, of course, are the result of abuse. Nonetheless, if significant suspicion exists in the physician's mind, the case must, by law, be reported to local Child Protective Social Services. If, in the physician's judgment, there is significant risk to returning the child to his home, social services may take emergency action and arrange temporary accommodation to ensure the child's safety.

A physician may have many reasons to suspect that a child has been sexually abused. These include unlikely physical signs or symptoms such as vaginal discharge or a torn hymenal ring in a young girl. The physician should be mindful that sexual abuse, while more common in girls, does happen to young boys. Recurrent abdominal pain, particularly if associated with constipation, encopresis or, in a girl, any vaginal symptoms, can be a sign of sexual abuse. If in the course of the evaluation other reasons for these symptoms cannot be identified, then it is worthwhile to ask questions about sexual abuse, such as, "Whenever I see this kind of a problem in a little girl, I wonder about the possibility of sexual abuse. Do you think this might be happening to your daughter?" The child can be asked directly, "Sometimes children who have pain like yours are worried because someone has been touching them in a way that they don't like. Has that been happening to you?" If the child appears reluctant to respond in front of a parent, consider talking with her privately.[15]

When suspected abuse is identified, it is important not only to report it to the local authorities, but also to involve a physician, social worker, or psychologist who specializes in childhood abuse. The total number of interviewers should be kept to a minimum, and it is usually not necessary for the primary physician to take an exhaustive history of the abuse. It is important, though, for the physician to clearly identify himself as an ally of the child and family and a resource person for any further questions that arise.

ENHANCING THE DOCTOR-PATIENT RELATIONSHIP

A common complaint that patients have about physicians is that they are distant and don't show genuine human concern for them or their families. This attitude, in and of itself, can inhibit patients' willingness to disclose what is really troubling them. Therefore it is important that physicians develop communication strategies that will enhance patient's self-disclosure.

Traditionally, physicians have been educated to maintain therapeutic distance by avoiding personal self-disclosure. Though this remains a controversial issue, there are a growing number of health professionals who advocate self-disclosure on the part of the clinician as a means of enhancing the genuineness of the doctor-patient relationship.[16] This may be particularly relevant in the context of the pediatric interview. A parent is likely to find reassurance when a doctor can share his or her own experience of caring for children, as a parent or otherwise. This challenge of humanizing the doctor-patient relationship while balancing the need for appropriate therapeutic distance is part of the art of medicine.

CONCLUSION

Talking with children and their parents can be one of the most enjoyable parts of a physician's practice of medicine. Helping children to become less fearful of doctors can be very satisfying. The American Academy of Pediatrics has concluded that families' discussions with physicians and the counseling they receive are the most important elements of child health care.[17] The pediatric interview is perhaps the most valuable tool physicians can use to assure the delivery of high-quality medical care to children. In these times of growing frustration with the dehumanization of medical care, physicians can reassure families by their willingness to listen and respond attentively to their concerns. As children grow older, the memory of comforting and engaging talks with their doctor will help them see physicians as their allies. When fear fades, new avenues to healing can be found.

REFERENCES

1. Ross, D., and S. Ross, "The Importance of Type of Question: Psychological Climate and Subject Set in Interviewing Children About Pain," *Pain*, 19:71–79, 1984.
2. Steward, M. S., K. Bussey, G. S. Goodman, and K. J. Saywitz, "Implications of Developmental Research for Interviewing Children," *Child Abuse and Neglect*, 17:25–37, 1993.
3. Korsch, B. M., E. K. Gozzi, and V. Francis, "Gaps in Doctor-Patient Communication. 1. Doctor-Patient Interaction and Patient Satisfaction," *Pediatrics*, 42:855–871, 1968.
4. Yudkin, S., "Six Children with Cough: The Second Diagnosis," *The Lancet*, II:561–563, September 9, 1961.
5. Tasem, M., B. Augenbraun, and S. L. Brown, "Family Group Interviewing with the Preschool Child and Both Parents," *Journal of American Child Psychiatry*, 4:330–340, 1965.
6. Liptak, G. S., B. S. Hulka, and J. C. Cassel, "Effectiveness of Physician-Mother Interactions During Infancy," *Pediatrics*, 60:186–192, 1977.
7. Bertakis, K. D., D. Roter, and S. M. Putnam, "The Relationship of Physician Interview Style to Patient Satisfaction," *Journal of Family Practice*, 32:175–181, 1991.
8. Hickson, G. B., W. A. Altemeier, and S. O'Connor, "Concerns of Mothers Seeking Care in Private Pediatric Offices: Opportunities for Expanding Services," *Pediatrics*, 72:619–624, 1983.
9. Starfield, B., and S. Barkowf, "Physicians' Recognition of Complaints Made by Parents About Their Children's Health," *Pediatrics*, 43:168–172, 1969.
10. Beckman, H. B., and R. M. Frankel, "The Effect of Physician Behavior on the Collection of Data," *Annals of Internal Medicine*, 101:692–696, 1984.
11. Rogers, J. C., and M. Rohrbaugh, "The SAGE-PAGE Trial: Do Family Genograms Make a Difference?" *Journal of American Board Family Practice*, 4:319–326, 1991.
12. Huygen, F., *The Medical Life History of Families*. Nijmejen, The Netherlands: Dekker and Van de Vegt, 1978.
13. Goldenring, J. M., and E. Cohen, "Getting into Adolescent Heads," *Contemporary Pediatrics*, July, 5:75–90, 1988.

14. Rakel, R. E., *Textbook of Family Practice*, Third Edition. Philadelphia: W. B. Saunders Co., 1984, p. 1240.
15. Leventhal, J. M., A. Bentovim, A. Elton, et al., "What to Ask When Sexual Abuse Is Suspected," *Archives Diseases of Children*, 62:1188–1195, 1987.
16. Young, R. C., "Rationale for Clinician Self-Disclosure and Research Agenda," *Image*, 20:196–199, 1988.
17. Reisinger, K. S., and J. A. Bires, "Anticipatory Guidance in Pediatrics," *Pediatrics*, 66:889–892, 1980.

7

INTERVIEWING THE FAMILY

KEY POINTS

1. Families affect the cause of illness and the outcome of treatment.
2. Clinicians can interview families in the hospital, office, nursing home, or home.
3. Families want more interviews from their physicians, especially at times of death or the diagnosis of serious illness.
4. Family discord may be seen with a patient who has multiple medical complaints.
5. The clinician should facilitate communication with members and not take sides with any member of the family.

Families play a major role in a person's health and illness. Recent studies have provided evidence that family support affects outcomes in heart attacks and a number of other conditions.[1] Illness frequently occurs at times of family crisis, and family members often call the clinician for explanations, advice, or reassurance. Those in primary care often find themselves discussing diagnostic findings and care plans with family members. Such contact is not limited to primary care but is common in the surgical fields and most other specialties. Virtually all clinicians need effective family interviewing skills to provide care that is comprehensive and compassionate.

There are many opportunities for contact with families in health care settings. Practitioners will encounter families at the bedside of hospitalized patients, a loved one may accompany the patient to an office visit, or a spouse may call ahead of a visit to make sure a certain problem is addressed. Indeed, if a clinician has not met with family members, it probably means that an opportunity to know more about the patient has been missed.

Patients usually appreciate it when their families are involved in major health decisions. In general, there is agreement among physicians and patients that family meetings are valuable when a family member is dying or has been hospitalized for a serious illness[2] (Table 7.1). However, physicians tend to underestimate the need at other times when their patients may consider such a meeting valuable.[3] Doherty and Baird have described five different levels at which a physician may choose to be involved in family-oriented care[4] (Table 7.2). Most experienced practitioners use the first two levels frequently. In one study family practice residents performed less well than in other aspects of patient care when addressing the meaning or implications of illness with patients and families.[5]

This chapter addresses the role of the family in illness, the impact of illness on the family, and strategies the clinician can use to obtain information from family meetings.

TABLE 7.1. Percentages of Patients Wanting
Family Conferences with Family Physician

Event	Percentage
Hospitalization for a serious illness	89
New diagnosis of a serious illness	83
Depression	71
Marital or relationship problems	48
Stress-related symptoms	49

TABLE 7.2. Five Levels of Physician Involvement with Families

1.	Minimal emphasis on families
2.	Ongoing medical information and advice
3.	Active dealings with feelings and support
4.	Systematic assessment and planned interventions
5.	Family therapy

TYPES OF FAMILIES

There are many types of families. While the most common stereotype of a family in the United States is that of the "nuclear family"—a father, mother, and children—such families have declined as a percentage of the population in the last few decades. The 1991 U.S. Census revealed that only 51 percent of families are the typical nuclear type. Clinicians today are likely to encounter families composed of single parents, gay or lesbian couples (sometimes with children), and extended families. Some "families" are not even related. A patient may consider his or her family to be a set of close friends who help with daily activities and shopping.

Extended families are commonly seen in certain minority groups and in immigrant populations. Grandparents, aunts and uncles, and cousins may live in the same household. There are a number of advantages to a large extended family, such as increased income and shared child care, but there may also be additional stresses. Examples of such stressors are competition for attention among family members and blurring lines of authority. Extended families may be closely knit, and the illness of any member will usually have an impact on all the others.

THE FAMILY LIFE CYCLE

Families that are together for some time go through a number of stages, each associated with specific stresses.[6] Members of the family may seek out health care workers at those times for advice or counsel. In these cases family interviewing can be used as a health maintenance tool. "Anticipatory guidance" can be given to family members about the kinds of stresses they may experience, or the physician can supply simple reassurance that their concerns are normal. The stages of the family life cycle are shown in Table 7.3.

Many families do not follow this same sequence of events. More couples are choosing to delay having children. Because divorce occurs so frequently, it might be considered an alternate phase of the family life cycle. Family members visit physicians more frequently around the time of divorce, and health problems are commonly seen at this time.[7]

TABLE 7.3. The Stages of the Family Life Cycle

Stage	Stress
Forming the family	New living situation Adjusting to partner's desires Adjusting to partner's family Finances
Birth of first child	Changes in work patterns Child-rearing Finances
Children in school	School performance Behavioral problems
Children leave home	Redefining parental roles Second career / mother's working
Retirement	Redefining self-worth More time together Adjusting to health problems Finances
Death	Bereavement Finances

FAMILY DYNAMICS

Every family has its own unique communication style, rules, alliances, belief systems, and ways of maintaining stability. While families can provide much support to one of its members during an illness, they may also play a part in its causation. Illness may cause great instability in one family, whereas in another family a similar illness can help stabilize a family in discord.

> Mr. Isenger suddenly developed epilepsy at age 59. A CAT scan of the brain revealed a tumor. All his life he had been a computer expert who maintained control over his family. His disease forced his wife to assume many of the household financial decisions, a job with which she was quite unaccustomed. Shortly thereafter she suffered a heart attack, having had no predisposing symptoms. Their daughter, a banker, then assumed responsibility for their financial affairs.

A common family rule is that one doesn't talk about family problems to strangers. Strangers may include health professionals. Such rules serve to maintain the equilibrium in the family. Equilibrium, or homeostasis, refers to the ability of the family to continue functioning even under difficult conditions. Hence, the principle of homeostasis may also be applied to a family in discord. In some families the fear of dissolving is greater than the fear of getting help from strangers.

Some members may form alliances with other family members for self-protection as a result of family rules limiting communication with outsiders, or as a way of maintaining equilibrium. A parent may align with a child for their mutual self-interest. This is commonly seen in alcoholic families. Alliances enable those in the family with less power to carry greater weight in decision making. Permanent alliances are often a sign of family discord and may decrease the family's ability to cope with problems.

Occasionally a particular member is blamed for all problems encountered by the family. Such "scapegoating" is another sign of family discord. Though scapegoating may be the first step in maintaining equilibrium, it inevitably leads to other problems. Strict authoritarian families run the highest risk for scapegoating. Because a child is often made the scapegoat, serious behavioral problems in the child may be the outcome.

THE CONCEPT OF FAMILY ILLNESS

Although most health care workers tend to view patients as isolated entities, the patients usually view themselves as members of families. When serious illness occurs, both the patient and the family must cope with the change in that person's health status. How the family will cope with an illness in one of its members can be analyzed by using a systems approach as illustrated in Figure 7.1. In this approach, each component of the system is intimately linked to all other components. Any process that affects one component will affect the others. Sometimes these effects will be strong, at other times minimal.

A systems approach suggests that the individual patient is a "symptom carrier" whose behavior, thoughts, physical state, and response to illness are influenced by his or her family as well as by the disease process itself.[8] One example of such a symptom carrier is the child with a behavior problem in school. Traditionally, the child is viewed as having a problem that needs correction. A family interview, however, might uncover the fact that this child is afraid to leave his mother at home alone because she is an alcoholic who falls frequently. His "behavioral problems" have allowed him to stay at home to care for his mother. He is thus the "identified patient" in this family system, but not the one who is most ill.

Families also tend to go through a predictable set of experiences when one member develops a serious illness. This normal process has been described as the "illness trajectory" by Burr and Good[9] (Table 7.4).

The first stage of this trajectory is the "onset of illness phase." It usually takes place before the diagnosis of a disease. If the illness is developing slowly, family members may notice changes in the patient's behavior or activities that cause concern. Depending on the family's communication style, these concerns may be discussed promptly or may

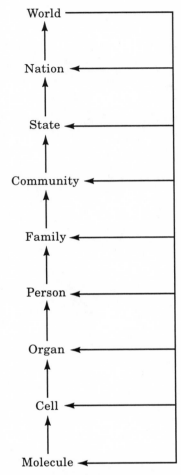

FIGURE 7.1. Systems Approach. Each component of the system interacts with all other components. A change in one part of the system will have some effect on the others.

TABLE 7.4. The Illness Trajectory

Phase	Key Tasks	Positive Family Behaviors	Problematic Behaviors
Onset of illness	Recognition of limits of health, willingness to accept care	Open questioning Offers of support	Denial of changes Blaming the victim
Impact of illness	Accepting the diagnosis, adjusting to physical capabilities, planning for treatment	Open discussion Sharing burden Supporting remaining capabilities	Destabilizing a dysfunctional milieau Abusive behaviors (drinking)
Initiation of therapy	Reorganization of responsibilities, managing financial and other implications	Shared responsibilities Realistic planning for the future	Children acting out (especially if the patient is the mother of young children)
Early recovery	Reintegration into the family and society	Flexible expectations New role assignments within family	Delayed reactions (particularly common when the illness was sudden and traumatic) Desires for secondary gain
Adjustment to permanency of outcome	Redefining self-worth and meaning	Acceptance of patient as they are	Unwillingness to accept or adjust to demands of the condition

Source: Adapted from Burr and Good. [9]

remain unspoken, causing increased anxiety in the patient. In the case of sudden onset of a disease (such as a myocardial infarction), this phase will be quite rapid. With many illnesses, such as emphysema, it will be more gradual and surrounded by uncertainty. During this time a family may seek the advice of clinicians about changes in the family member with whom they are concerned. They may label the patient a "complainer" because the disease has not advanced enough to cause outright illness, but rather a change in the patient's physical or emotional responses. As the problem progresses, however, diagnosis usually becomes clear.

The second stage is the "impact phase." The moment of being told the diagnosis is often clearly remembered by the patient. The patient may become depressed or withdrawn, and the family may cope with the patient's response through denial. How well the patient adjusts to the illness is greatly influenced by the way in which the family responds. Some families encourage open discussion of feelings and plans for dealing with the illness. These families may actually become stronger as a result of the illness. Others, usually those families that were having difficulties before the illness, will become dysfunctional when a family member becomes ill. The additional strain on the family communication may upset a delicate balance and thus have a disruptive effect.

The "therapeutic phase" then follows. The impact on the family will depend on which family member is hospitalized. When mothers of smaller children are hospitalized, there is a high risk of family disorganization, creating discomfort for all. When children are hospitalized, the child may experience feelings of abandonment, while parents may feel guilty over not having "protected" their youngster from illness. Though usually irrational, these feelings affect the way the family copes with the illness and influence decisions they make regarding treatment. Such feelings certainly affect their relations with health care professionals involved in the patient's care.

A 75-year-old man was admitted to the hospital for severe pneumonia. He had had a number of strokes and his ability to swallow had been affected, leading to decreased oral intake and weight loss. Before admission he had lived in an adult foster home. Because he was unable to give informed consent as to whether he should receive endotracheal intubation, his daughter was called. But she had been estranged from him for two years. When she saw his gaunt appearance she immediately blamed his caregiver at the foster home. She said she wanted "everything done for him because he's obviously been mistreated." But when his swallowing problems and history of strokes were explained, she began to cry and said, "I don't know what you should do. I guess I just feel guilty for not visiting him for the last two years."

The family goes through the "early recovery phase" as treatment progresses. Many experience an unanticipated letdown, a delayed reaction to the stress of the illness, during this time. The patient, particularly if he or she is a child, may cling to the illness, even when improvement is seen. The patient may be receiving some secondary gain such as increased attention. This is often seen in families that were in a state of discord, like that resulting from marital problems, before the child became ill. The parents may be so involved in the care of the child that they temporarily put aside their differences and argue less. The child may then unconsciously wish to remain ill to keep the parents together.

Finally, the patient either recovers or must adapt to having a chronic disease. This phase is the "adjustment to permanency of outcome." The clinician must continue to be aware that unwillingness to adjust to the reality of the illness may be a sign of family discord. In this case, as well as during the impact and early recovery phases, family conferences can be extremely important in resolving the difficulties. Awareness of these phases of a family's experience with illness will help the clinician provide anticipatory counseling and advice.

SITES FOR FAMILY INTERVIEWS

Most clinicians see the hospital as the main site for family interviews. Indeed, discussions with the patient's family are usually a critical part of the hospital care. Opportunities for such discussions abound. Key times when family discussions can be most helpful include:

1. During the diagnostic phase. Particularly in the case of the very young or very old, corroboration of information is often needed.
2. Explaining the diagnosis. Especially with life-threatening illnesses such as heart attacks, cancer, or chronic illness such as dementia, family involvement will be needed. [10]
3. Discussing treatment options. Adherence to medication regimens is often enhanced when family members are involved. When the treatment entails ongoing discomfort for the patient (e.g., surgery, special diets, or chemotherapy), a family conference is particularly helpful. [11,12]
4. Predischarge planning. Summarizing the findings, treatments, and recommendations for follow-up helps the patient and family carry through with medical plans.

There are some drawbacks to the hospital as an interview site. The patient and family are on the clinician's "turf" and may feel inhibited about disclosing information or expressing concerns. Children may be excluded unnecessarily by restrictive visiting hours. Family members often visit the patient in the evening, and clinicians interested in family interviews may need to schedule special afternoon or evening sessions.

The office and clinic are appropriate sites for a family interview. Visits can be scheduled at the end of the day when more time is available. The limiting factor is having a conference room large enough for all family members to be present.

Should the patient reside in a nursing home, a family conference can be held at the patient's bedside or in a larger meeting room there. These patients may feel very lonely. A family interview affords them attention and gives the clinician a chance to gain useful historical information.

Finally, the patient's home should not be forgotten as an excellent site for family interviews. Here the patient and the family are on their own turf. It is the clinician who is the visitor. The most accurate picture of family interaction is seen in the home. The family's capacity to provide care can be observed and direct suggestions can be made.

THE FAMILY INTERVIEW IN MEDICAL CARE

Acute Health Crises

When a patient has been newly diagnosed with a serious illness, a family interview is indicated. The best times for the interview are either shortly after the diagnosis has been made or before discharge from the hospital. The latter gives the patient enough time to be free of the effects of the anesthetic agents or simply to let the diagnosis "sink in." It also allows adequate time before the patient goes home to answer questions and make plans for the future. Patients with heart attacks, strokes, or cancer and their families should certainly be given this opportunity. Most families are quite willing to adjust their schedules to meet the needs of the clinician if enough advance warning is given. Other, less serious problems can also be addressed in a family interview. Any discussion of sexual problems should eventually include the patient's partner. Behavioral problems in children usually can only be resolved with adequate family involvement.

The death of any family member creates the greatest stress for a family.[13] Deaths that occur in hospitals are particularly stressful. Hospice programs have pioneered the use of bereavement groups to help families adjust to the loss of their loved one.

Finally, the diagnosis of an inherited disorder (such as sickle-cell anemia or Tay-Sachs disease) usually leads to a family interview. While obtaining an accurate genetic history is one goal of this meeting, the family's emotional responses and their concerns about future pregnancies should also be discussed. Options for later treatment can be discussed as well.

Health Care in Chronic Illness

Because changes in the health status of a person with a chronic illness are less dramatic than in acute illness, the need for family interviews may be underestimated. There are, however, many circumstances in which a family conference can be useful. The patient who is not responding to therapy may be having difficulty in complying with the treatment regimen. When the family is anticipating institutionalization of an older person, a family meeting is essential. It provides an opportunity to assess the need for such a change more accurately as well as to deal with the guilt feelings commonly experienced by family members.

When a patient's desire for further interventions is being discussed (e.g., cardiopulmonary resuscitation, living wills, advanced directives), the involvement of family ensures that they have heard—and hopefully understand—the patient's wishes. It also helps the patient feel less alone and fearful.

Diagnostic and Treatment Dilemmas

Family meetings are very helpful in the case of the patient who represents a diagnostic or treatment dilemma. The patient whose "tests are all normal," or who has persistently asked many doctors, "Why can't any of you find the problem?" often has a family problem that is being masked by the illness.

A 58-year-old woman complained of constant left facial pain of seven years' duration. Complete work-ups, including special X-rays, revealed no cause. Relaxation, medication, acupuncture, electrical stimulation, and drugs all gave no relief.

An interview with the family revealed that the patient was dissatisfied with her relationship with her husband, who was 58 years old. She took satisfaction in life only when her adult daughters came over to take her to one of her many doctors' appointments.

During the family interview the patient was instructed to communicate her "medical worries" only to the physician, not to her daughters. The daughters were instructed to spend the same amount of time they had been giving to taking their mother to doctors' appointments to shopping or dining with her. The patient's pains gradually disappeared.

Family Interviews in Managed Care

While concerns about time constraints may lead some to forgo family interviews in a managed care environment, capitated medical care plans actually may offer greater flexibility in planning visits. This is because the burden of needing a "diagnosis" to justify the visit for reimbursement is lessened. Family visits can be viewed as "health promotion" activities, which managed care typically views positively. A well-timed family visit may lead to fewer visits later, thereby meeting the requirements of cost-effective care. However, it will still be the role of the care provider to recognize the need and advocate for the use of family visits in this new care setting.

CONDUCTING A FAMILY INTERVIEW

Convening the Family Members

In hospital settings the family interview can be convened easily by speaking with the patient about the need for such a meeting. Occasionally, as in the case of a comatose patient or a child, the spouse or parent will need to be contacted. It is important to have the patient's permission so as not to undermine the clinician-patient relationship. Once permission has been gained, it must be decided who would be the most appropriate person to contact other family members. Usually this can be done by the patient, but the authority of the physician can be used to gather the family together, particularly when the family is disengaged or very distraught as a result of the patient's illness.

In some larger families various members may contact health care workers individually. This is time-consuming and may lead to distortion of information learned secondhand. When this occurs, a remark by the clinician such as, "I've now spoken with several members of your family and would like to meet with all of you together to summarize the information we have so far and to give you an opportunity to ask any questions," will serve to set up the first interview.

In outpatient settings a time should be scheduled when the entire family can meet. Obviously, it is best to have a meeting room that will accommodate all family members. The clinician should observe the early interaction of the various members as the meeting begins. Where do they choose to sit? Does one person "take charge" at the meeting? How do parents manage children's activities and questions? Are there any obvious alliances among members?

Only in rare instances should the patient be excluded from the interview. For instance, a patient with severe communication difficulties (as after a stroke) might not be able to follow the conversation, leading to increased anxiety. Even in these cases, the clinician and the family should meet with the patient afterward to share basic information discussed.

Opening the Interview

There are several ways to open a family interview. The choice will depend on the reason for the meeting. If the original purpose of a family meeting is to discuss diagnostic findings, these should simply be stated. If the goal of the session is to discuss treatment options, then more open-ended probing of the patient's and family members' feelings is in order. In general, it is important to begin interviews in an open-ended fashion because the clinician's concerns may not be the same as the family's.

> Mary Perera recently had a computed tomography scan of the abdomen that revealed massively enlarged lymph nodes. She feels reasonably well. She wants to have her family involved in the treatment decisions.
>
> DOCTOR: Mary has told me that she shared with you the results of her X-ray. What questions would you like to ask me?

This type of opening is neutral enough to allow a wide variety of questions from clarifying the diagnosis (since the patient may not have transmitted that information accurately) to discussing the various treatment options. Family members may also ask questions about the cause of the illness or their role in ongoing care. Since the entire family is hearing the clinician's words together, there is less chance of misunderstanding.

It is often helpful to convene families not only to transmit diagnostic information but also to help them cope with the feelings generated by the diagnosis of a life-threatening illness.

> Seldon Smith is recovering from a heart attack. He has often expressed how irritated he is with his family because "they are all treating me as if I was fine china that would break if they touched me."

NURSE: I asked you all to meet together because, in my experience, most families have a lot of questions about how they should treat their loved one after a heart attack. How about you?

Here the clinician helps the family discuss the problem openly and can dispel some of the common myths held by lay persons, such as the notion that all heart attack patients are fragile.

Some families have strong disagreements about treatment plans. A group interview serves to help families make decisions together about these difficult problems.

Ms. Perera is considering not having a surgical procedure to diagnose the cause of her enlarged lymph nodes, as her doctor had advised. Her husband wants her to try faith healing. Her daughter thinks she ought to have the surgery.

DOCTOR: Mary is facing a very difficult decision about whether or not to have surgery. What do each of you think about that?

Although the clinician may have strong opinions about the best treatment, patients' decisions are influenced by a variety of advisors. A high value is usually placed on their family members' thoughts. The above opening gives the clinician an opportunity to see how the family solves problems in addition to getting different family members' opinions. The process of problem solving will allow the clinician to observe the family roles and to develop plans for later work with the family. Families that have difficulty reaching consensus about such problems may do so because of the stress of the situation. However, their difficulty may also be evidence of pre-existing family discord. In that case the health crisis may provide an opportunity to identify a family's need for therapy. Appropriate referrals can then be made.

Eliciting Information

The next stage of the interview is eliciting more information. With some families, particularly those that are accustomed to open exchanges of feelings, this is easily accomplished. Such families will still need an interviewer to facilitate the more quiet members to participate.

Ms. Patrick, a woman with multiple medical complaints, was asked to bring her family in to discuss the results of a comprehensive diagnostic study. Her husband and daughter attended the interview. After the clinician opened the interview, the daughter spent much time inquiring about details of the examination. The husband was essentially silent.

NURSE: Mr. Patrick, I notice you've been pretty quiet while the rest of your family has been doing most of the questioning? Do you have any questions?

MR. PATRICK (*angrily*): Yeah, I'd like to know when she's going to be well again so our life can get back to normal.

Another method of eliciting information about how the family is functioning is to comment on the process of communication in the interview. Families have well-practiced communication styles and can sometimes discuss a matter extensively without really getting to the heart of it. Commenting about how they are communicating, rather than just addressing what they are discussing, helps them move to a different level of interaction.

The Chase family was actively discussing whether their senior member should come home from the hospital after a serious illness or go to a nursing home. Sarah Chase, the patient's daughter, who would be caring for her, brought up a number of concerns about the option of home care. The rest of the family dismissed the daughter's concerns with little or no discussion.

INTERVIEWER: I've noticed that each time Ms. Chase brings up a concern about her mother coming home, the rest of you seem to dismiss it.

Some families have a difficult time discussing an issue openly, honestly, and thoroughly. One person, often the father, may dominate the discussion. In these situations the best approach is to guide the discussion away from the facts and to call attention to the process of discussing them. Calling attention to the lack of participation by family members other than the controlling member may open up the discussion, and it may even help the family learn to communicate better.

It is extremely important not to take sides with particular family members. This kind of alliance will destroy the other family members' trust in the clinician and limit effective interventions. When a family is having a heated argument, one member may ask the clinician to decide for them. It is best to avoid doing so. Any answer is unlikely to be the right one for all members of the family and will only lead to further conflict. One approach to this situations is exemplified in the next example:

> Mr. Roberts had been hospitalized recently. Some of his children wanted him to stop driving because his reflexes were too slow. One daughter asked the physician to "tell him he can't drive anymore." His son then said that if he can't drive, "He'll just die."
>
> DOCTOR: I can see that you disagree about your father's driving after he is discharged from the hospital. Let's discuss this question with him. I think he should hear about your concern for his safety as well as his independence.

This kind of statement identifies the concerns of both children without taking sides. It also clarifies the role of the clinician as patient advocate. Finally, it should help the family work out their problems together.

Clarifying Content

Family members often have hidden fears and concerns that need to be addressed. One is a sense of guilt about the cause of the illness or accident. This is particularly characteristic of parents of young children. While some parents may be open about their concerns regarding their role in the illness, many are not. Others may present a deluge of questions, often repeating the same or similar ones. Some parents may appear to be more distressed than would be expected given the degree of the illness. Feelings of guilt about one's role in the development of an illness are not limited to parents of children. For instance, spouses of alcoholics often believe they could have prevented the alcoholic from drinking. Whenever family members share their love for one person, they are likely to feel some responsibility for that individual's health.

The nurse, after cleansing a boy's badly bruised leg that resulted from a fall from a bicycle, noticed that the boy's father appeared to be angry with his wife.

NURSE: Mr. Kyle, you look a little irritated.

MR. KYLE: Well, I've told my wife not to let Paul ride that bike. Now look what's happened.

NURSE: Mrs. Kyle, how do you feel about the accident?

By asking this question, the nurse helps the family talk out the problem without taking sides. She also does not give reassurance too soon (i.e., by saying, "Oh, no, accidents will happen"). Children's accidents happen more frequently during times of family stress, so ensuing discussion may help to prevent further calamities.[14] Many other problems may be lurking behind the obvious medical issues. Concerns about changes in the roles of the family members, possible financial burdens of care, and fear of transmission of disease may be in the family members' minds. These can be elicited by asking, "What other concerns or questions would you like to discuss before we wrap it up?"

CONCLUSION

Because our society is composed of "families"—families of origin, extended families, families of friends—many individuals are affected when one person becomes ill. The family can help the patient recover from illness, but it may also prolong or even prevent recovery. By using family interviewing skills, the clinician can help families cope with the emotional and other burdens created by illness. According to an old Chinese saying, "Crisis equals danger plus opportunity." In a health care crisis, the clinician may have an opportunity to help a troubled family.

REFERENCES

1. Case, R. B., A. J. Moss, N. Case, et al., "Living Alone after Myocardial Infarction: Impact on Prognosis," *Journal of the American Medical Association*, 267:515–519, 1992.

2. Kushner, K., D. Meyer, and J. P. Hansen, "Patients' Attitudes toward Physician Involvement in Family Conferences," *Journal of Family Practice*, 28:73–78, 1989.

3. Kushner, K., and D. Meyer, "Family Physicians' Perceptions of the Family Conference," *Journal of Family Practice*, 28:65–68, 1989.

4. Doherty, W., M. A. Baird, *Family Centered Medical Care: A Clinical Casebook*. New York: Guilford Press, 1987.

5. Shapiro, J., and D. D. Schiermer, "Resident Psychosocial Performance: A Brief Report," *Journal of Family Practice*, 8:10–13, 1991.

6. Rolland, J. S., "The Family Impact of Illness and Disability." In *Essentials of Family Medicine*, R. E. Rakel (ed.). Philadelphia: W. B. Saunders, 1993. pp. 49–66.

7. Verbrugge, L. M., "Marital Status and Health," *Journal of Marriage and the Family*, 41:267–285, 1979.

8. Bateson, G., *Steps to an Ecology of Mind*. New York: Ballantine Books, 1972.

9. Burr, B., and B. Good, "The Impact of Illness on the Family." In *Family Medicine*, R. Rakel (ed.). New York: Springer-Verlag, 1978. p. 228.

10. Reifler, B. V., and S. Wu, "Managing Families of the Demented Elderly," *Journal of Family Practice*, 6:1051–1056, 1982.

11. Morisky, D. E., D. M. Levine, L. W. Green, et al., "Five Year Blood Pressure Control and Mortality Following Health Education for Hypertensive Patients," *American Journal of Public Health*, 73:153–162, 1983.

12. Pearce, J. W., and O. J. LeBow, "Role of Spouse Involvement in the Behavioral Treatment of Overweight Women," *Journal of Consulting Clinical Psychology*, 49:236–244, 1981.

13. Clayton, P., "Mortality and Morbidity in the First Year of Widowhood," *Archives of General Psychiatry*, 30:747–750, 1974.

14. Huygen, F., *Family Medicine: The Medical Life History of Families*. Nijmejen, The Netherlands: Dekker and Van de Vegt, 1978.

8

INTERVIEWING THE OLDER ADULT

KEY POINTS

1. Be careful not to let negative attitudes toward the aged affect the interview.
2. Pay attention to sensory deficits, such as hearing and vision, that could adversely affect the interview.
3. Older persons may be sensitive about discussing personal or psychological issues.
4. Assessment of the patient's social support system and mental status are important components of the interview.
5. It is the clinician's job to broach the subjects of sexuality, substance abuse, and advanced directives.

The population of those over the age of 65 in the United States is increasingly rapidly. While 13 percent of the general population is over 65 today, it is predicted that by the year 2020 that figure will rise to over 20 percent. People are living longer and fewer people are dying at younger ages. The complexion of our society is changing as a result. In primary care and in specialty settings the age profile of physicians' practices is advancing. Health professionals of all types will be spending more time caring for older persons.

Illness is much more common in older persons, though many older people live very healthy lives and rarely see a physician. In general, though, elderly persons use health care services at three times the rate of younger persons. The older patient often has multiple chronic medical problems, such as hypertension, diabetes, arthritis, and heart failure. When acute illness occurs, it is often superimposed on a long-standing disorder.

From the viewpoint of the older person, concerns about diseases are usually secondary to worries about functional disabilities. Loss of the ability to live independently is one of the greatest fears of older people. Many geriatric patients have greater fear of becoming dependent on others or a burden on their family than of death itself. Unfortunately, much medical treatment is devoted to the management of disease rather than the enhancement of function.

Although 80 percent of the population over age 65 have at least one chronic disorder, from vision impairment to heart disease, older people are remarkably adaptable. When asked to rate their personal health, for example, 85 percent reported being in good or excellent health.[1] While this figure probably reflects some denial, it also clearly indicates that the mere presence of a disease is not enough to make most older people see themselves as unwell. To assist the older person in coping with chronic disease, the physician needs excellent interviewing skills to best understand how to help.

Because of the high prevalence of multiple medical and functional problems, the fact that as people age they become more physiologically diverse, and the frequent pressure of differences in values and life experiences between the patient and the interviewer, effective interviewing skills and an accurate history play a crucial role in care of the elderly patient.

Managed care places an additional burden in caring for older persons when there are expectations for shorter visits. Efficient, high-quality interviewing skills become even more important in these settings. However, most managed care plans also recognize that the care of frail, older adults requires more time, and so they allow for longer or more frequent visits. These programs are aware that the sense of being rushed by the doctor often leads the patient to lose satisfaction with their care and may provoke the patient to choose another health care plan. This chapter deals with the process of interviewing the aged, unique aspects of the content of such interviews, and some of the common problems encountered.

THE PROCESS OF THE INTERVIEW

With older patients, the physical setting is an important factor in conducting a succcsssful interview. Older patients often have deficits in vision and hearing, so attention to these details will facilitate communication.[2]

Hearing and Vision

The room light should clearly illuminate the interviewer's face so that lip reading can be accomplished if necessary. A quiet room without extraneous noises is very important when interviewing patients with hearing aids as all sounds tend to be amplified equally. Older patients may hear more when seated in the corner because sounds are magnified. Speaking clearly, slowly, and distinctly is appreciated, but the volume of one's voice should be raised only if necessary. Some older persons may be offended if the voice is raised without need.

Many older persons may be unaware of or unwilling to admit their hearing problems. These patients do not use hearing aids. Communication with such patients can be made much easier by the use of a handheld amplifier. The interviewer speaks into a small microphone-amplifier, about the size of a beeper, and the patient wears small headphones similar to the type used for personal cassette players. Such an instrument can make an interview in a busy clinic or hospital ward much more private.

If the patient wears dentures, they should be in place. Embarrassment is a definite deterrent to open communication. Communication of certain words is more difficult without the dentures and recognition of the patient's nonverbal facial cues can be affected.

Beginning the Interview

It is extremely important that the clinician introduce himself or herself at the beginning. Older people grew up in a time when propriety and decorum were held in great esteem. Many older persons harbor apprehension about the medical profession, and politeness helps to set the patient at ease. Most older people prefer to be addressed by their surnames rather than first names.

Once these measures have been taken, the interview can proceed. As with other patients, one should begin with open-ended questions. Most older patients will be able to respond without difficulty to this type of questioning, and in these cases the techniques used do not differ significantly from those discussed in Chapter 2. Many physicians immediately begin a series of highly specific questions when talking with older patients, perhaps because they are concerned that it will take too much time cover all the patient's problems.[3] If patients react negatively to this type of questioning, it can have a deleterious effect on their satisfaction with their health care.[4] Physicians are often evaluated by their communication skills rather than their technical expertise.

Some elderly patients are frightened when being interviewed. They may fear institutionalization or hospitalization. They may have some memory problems, and the anticipation of an embarrassing discovery of their memory loss may inhibit their ability to communicate. Many older patients have been in medical settings numerous times. They are "experienced" patients and have often been "trained" to give their history in response to a short question-and-answer format. These patients may be uneasy with an open-ended line of inquiry. It then becomes important to discern the reason for their difficulty. If a patient is not responsive to questions, it is wise to focus on the process of the interview rather than to try to convince the patient of the need to answer questions.

> An 85-year-old woman was being interviewed by a second-year medical student. The student began the interview by asking, "What sort of problems are you having?" The patient responded angrily, "You're the doctor; you tell me." The student answered, "You sound upset." The patient then admitted, "Well, wouldn't you be if your daughter just told you that you have to go into a nursing home?"

Discussing Personal Issues

Some older patients have difficulty responding to questions that pertain to feelings or psychological issues. Many were raised in a social climate in which personal problems were not discussed, sometimes not even within the family. They may also be less likely to open up early in the interview, waiting instead until they feel they can trust the interviewer. If reassurance or a gentle confrontation that this line of questioning appears to be difficult for the patient does not restore the flow of communication, it is best to summarize and move on.

> CLINICIAN: So you lost your husband twelve years ago. What was that like for you?
> PATIENT: I don't like to talk about it actually. (*Silence.*)
> CLINICIAN: I can see this is hard for you to talk about.
> PATIENT: Well, it sort of brings up bad memories.
> CLINICIAN: Bad memories?
> PATIENT: Yes. But what about my heart? Am I going to have to take that new medicine?
> CLINICIAN: Well, when you care to talk about it, I really would like to hear about the death of your husband. As to your medicine . . .

Reminiscence

Clinicians are often concerned that the older patient will go off on a tangent and begin telling long stories. This common habit, called reminiscence, helps them integrate their previous experiences into the present. However, it may also be evidence of some intellectual impairment, particularly if excessive. Patients with memory problems will "reminisce" because they cannot converse in the here-and-now. Pathological reminiscing is usually tangential and not associated with the discussion at hand. A simple question such as, "And how does that relate to what we were discussing?" will get the loquacious patient back on track. Such a question is partly diagnostic because if the patient cannot get back to the previous discussion, this may indicate underlying memory problems.[5] The clinician must decide whether or not to interrupt the patient, based on the estimated value of the patient's reminiscence and the time available to the clinician.

Pacing

The pacing in an interview is referred to as tempo, and the interviewing tempo is different with older patients, tending to be slower. The speed of responses to both nonverbal tasks and verbal questions declines with age. Older patients are less likely to take risks and less willing to make errors than younger patients,[6] hence they may "cogitate" over a question before answering. Persons with serious illnesses may not have the physical stamina for a long and detailed interview. Those who are frail may need to have the interview completed on a second visit.

Including Family Members and Friends in Interviews

Eighty-five percent of all care provided to frail elders is supplied by family and friends. About 20 percent of those over age 70 have memory problems and are unable to give an accurate history. Therefore, it is important to consider whether a family member should also be interviewed when an older patient is seen. In our society, it is usually daughters or daughters-in-law who are the primary caregivers to older relatives.[7] These caregivers may provide quite a different picture than that presented by the patient.

> During the interview, a 75-year-old man carefully described his daily activities: working in his garden, going for a walk with his dog in the afternoon, and reading extensively. When his daughter was interviewed later, she reported that although he had a large garden in the past, he had been housebound for the last three years due to Alzheimer's disease and only left home for visits to the doctor. He still thumbed through cherished books but was unable to remember what he read.

Some very old patients have outlived all their family members and depend on friends for everything from social activities to help with daily activities. Such friends will often accompany the patient to a hospital or

TABLE 8.1. Promoting an Effective
Interview with Older Persons

1. Pay attention to sensory deficits
2. Allow adequate time
3. Allow reasonable reminiscence
4. Involve family and friends
5. Slow the pace of the interview

office in times of distress. Patients should be asked if they wish to include their friends in the interview.

In summary, though the process of interviewing older adults is usually very similar to that of interviewing younger patients, certain adjustments must often be made (Table 8.1). Attention to sensory deficits that affect communication is needed. Allowing time to reminisce may help the older person integrate past medical experiences into the present. Avoiding rapid-fire questioning and allowing for slower response time will decrease both the patient's and the clinician's frustration. Finally, viewing the patient as a member of a family or other support system helps the interviewer understand the patient as a whole person.

THE CONTENT OF THE INTERVIEW

The main content areas of the interview of an older person are the same as with any other patient. Certain areas play a larger role (Table 8.2). An important difference is the large role of the patient's social supports in maintaining health and in coping with disease. The past medical history is usually much more extensive. Because independence is so valued by older persons (since they fear its loss), the review of systems should include specific questions about the patient's ability to perform daily activities and the presence of common geriatric conditions. An important area to examine is mental functioning. Finally, the interviewer is responsible for bringing up subjects that are very imporant to the older person but often difficult to discuss, such as sexuality, substance abuse, and advanced planning for life-sustaining treatment.

TABLE 8.2. Important Components in the Geriatric Interview

Content	Differences
Patient profile	Assess social support systems
	Use of community resources
Past medical history	More extensive
	Multiple medical conditions
	Multiple surgeries
Medication review	Multiple medications
	Multiple prescribers
	Over-the-counter medications
Review of systems	Activities of Daily Living (ADL)
	Common geriatric conditions (falls, incontinence, etc.)
Mental functioning	Standardized question
	Standardized assessment tool
Difficult subjects	Sexuality
	Drugs and alcohol
	Advanced planning for life-sustaining treatments

Patient Profile

Social supports are usually divided into informal (family and friends) and formal (paid workers) (Table 8.3). Although elderly persons often suffer multiple medical problems, those who do not have a strong support system are likely to do less well when ill. Patients with limited social supports are more likely to become residents of long-term care institutions. Furthermore, their dependence on social support systems is largely influenced by their ability to care for themselves.

This topic can be directly approached if it has not arisen spontaneously. A simple question like, "Who helps you out if there are times you cannot take care of all you have to do by yourself?" will promote a discussion of the patient's support system. Usually the main sources of informal support are the spouse, the daughter, or the daughter-in-law. The older person should be questioned about involvement in church groups, senior citizen centers, day-care centers, or other social activities. Hobbies and volunteer work can be a positive factor in adjusting to retirement. Pets tend to increase an older person's sense of responsibility and companionship.

Because many elderly persons survive on fixed incomes, knowledge of their living arrangements is helpful. Does the area have a high crime rate? Is the house safe as far as locks and exits are concerned? What is the patient's income? Obviously, those living on Social Security may have difficulty following a health professional's recommendations if the costs are too high. Medications are not covered by Medicare, and poorer patients may have to choose between paying rent and refilling prescriptions.

Past Medical History

The past medical history of an older person can be quite extensive. Multiple medical problems and past operations are a common pattern. How can all this information be managed? An emphasis on how any problem in the past may affect the patient's present-day functioning will help to keep the past medical information in perspective. Except for rheumatic fever, for instance, childhood illnesses are unlikely to affect the older patient at present. But in the patient with a recent stroke the past history of high blood pressure or diabetes is likely to be of considerable importance. The patient's present condition should lead the clinician in his or her pursuit of the past history.

A form, completed by the patient, containing a checklist of past medical and surgical problems will save time and allow more attention to be given to the patient during the interview. Having the patient bring old medical records from previous physicians provides details about past

TABLE 8.3. Types of Social Support Systems

Informal	Formal
Family members	Home health aides
Neighbors	Live-in attendants
Friends	Visiting nurses association
Church members	Meals-on-Wheels

diagnoses and medications used as well as previously performed diagnostic tests.

Medications

Approximately 85 percent of older people are on at least one prescription drug. Virtually all regularly take at least one over-the-counter drug. The risk of overmedication and adverse drug reactions is greatly magnified by the multiple use. Thus, it is essential to ascertain all the patient's present medications and as many of the past ones as can be remembered. Sometimes it is best to have patients bring in a bag of all their medications for review. They should be advised to look not only in the medicine cabinet, but also the bedside table, the kitchen cupboard, and the side table of the chair in which they watch television. A helpful way to assess patients' knowledge of their medications is to hold up the bottle (or show them one of the pills in the bottle) and ask, "And how often do you take this one?"

Review of Systems

The variability of physiologic function from individual to individual increases with age. There is also more variability in the activities of daily living (ADL), those functions that one must perform in order to live independently. Bathing, preparing and consuming food, toileting, walking, and dressing are taken for granted by most younger people. Limitations in any of these areas can be a severe deterrent to independence, and such limitations occur more frequently as people age. Most persons over age 75 have some deficit in independent living skills.[7]

These activities are best assessed by asking patients to describe the last few meals prepared, by watching them remove a sweater or shirt before the physical exam, and by observing them as they get out of a chair or walk down the hall. A standard series of questions has been developed to survey the patient's perception of independence (Table 8.4):

TABLE 8.4. Brief Screening Questions for Functional Activities

Functional History: Activities of Daily Living ("B-A-T-T-E-D")
Do you have any trouble with: (If answer is "no," ask "How do you do it?"
Score "yes" if help is needed.)

1. Bathing?	Yes_____	No_____
2. Walking (Ambulation)?	Yes_____	No_____
3. Making Transfers?	Yes_____	No_____
4. Using the Toilet?	Yes_____	No_____
5. Eating?	Yes_____	No_____
6. Dressing?	Yes_____	No_____

Instrumental Activities of Daily Living ("S-C-U-M-M")

7. Shopping?	Yes_____	No_____
8. Cooking or Cleaning?	Yes_____	No_____
9. Using Transportation?	Yes_____	No_____
10. Managing Money?	Yes_____	No_____
11. Managing Medications?	Yes_____	No_____

CLINICIAN: Do you have any trouble with bathing?
PATIENT: No.
CLINICIAN: How do you do it?
PATIENT: I don't take baths, I just lean up against the sink and splash myself. If I tried to get down in the tub I'd never get back up again.

Any activity that has been reported by the patient but not observed by the interviewer may need to be substantiated by other family members if the clinician has reason to doubt the patient's account.

Certain conditions are common in geriatric patients. Often these conditions are accepted by the patient or family as being "due to old age," and an opportunity to treat the problem is missed. Therefore, it is incumbent upon the clinician to bring up these subjects. Urinary incontinence affects about 10 to 20 percent of community-dwelling elders.[8] Embarrassment may prevent them from mentioning this symptom. About a third of elders fall in the home each year.[9] Depression is common in old age, [10] and sometimes health-care providers fail to detect it. Formal standardized tests, such as the Geriatric Depression Scale, [11] have been developed for use during an interview. However, the simple question, "Do you often feel sad or depressed?" will help identify those patients who need more in-depth assessment. [12]

Mental Status Examination

Only 5 percent of the population over the age of 65 suffers from dementia, or cognitive impairment. However, approximately 20 percent of those over 80 have this disorder, which was formerly called "senility." Such patients are well represented in health care settings. Cognitive impairment is a significant deterrent to independent living. It is crucial that it be recognized and that reversible causes be detected before the patient is labeled with the diagnosis of a permanent and progressive disorder.

Surprisingly, health care providers commonly fail to recognize patients with dementia. This is because in the earlier stages of dementia patients rely on old memories and communication patterns, ones that are well established and not likely to be affected until later in the course of the disease. The patient may be affable and able to carry on a conversation without apparent difficulty. It is only when the patient's memory is actually tested that the cognitive impairment is discovered.

A 79-year-old woman was interviewed by a nurse practitioner in a geriatric clinic. The patient described her home in honest terms, saying that since her husband had died she really didn't keep her house as clean as she used to. She preferred to spend her time gardening and reported raising three varieties of orchids. She spoke freely and did not exhibit any unusual uneasiness during the interview. Upon specific questioning, however, she was unsure about the date and could not remember her address or her age.

The mental status exam is an objective measurement of cognitive function that should supplement, not replace, the subjective data gleaned during the interview.[13] The Mini-Mental Status Exam is a series of questions that are administered to the patient.[14] A total of 30 points is possible. Normal persons usually score 28 or greater. A score below 24 is cause for concern. The test can be given in about ten minutes and can be repeated over time to assess changes in cognitive function (Fig. 8.1).

It is important to put the patient at ease before administering the test. It can be introduced as "another method of evaluating your health, like the physical exam." The interviewer may wish to add, "Although some of these questions may seem simple and others hard, they will help me to select the best treatment for you." If a patient shows some exasperation with failure during the test, he or she should be encouraged to continue after a supportive comment about the difficulty. It is not necessary to correct all mistakes made by the patient; in fact, doing so may cause the patient to perform more poorly. A discussion of the patient's general performance is likely to be appreciated, however, especially if the goal is to attempt to improve a problem about which the patient has already expressed concern.

In scoring the Mini-Mental Status Exam, the clinician should note each answer and not give the patient the benefit of the doubt by excusing a mistake. If scoring is consistent, the scores can be used over time to measure changes in function. Hence, it is important to use a standardized scoring method. One can interpret the scores more liberally. For instance, the patient who scores only two on the data section (missing the date, day of the week, and month) may be excused for these errors if he has recently woken up from a week-long coma that began at the end of the month. Some patients will not be able to reach a full score of 30 points because of blindness (unable to read instructions and draw the figure) or illiteracy. Their scores should then be assessed with these factors in mind.

Family History

The family history, like the past medical history, can be extensive with older patients. The use of a family genogram, drawn with the patient

1. Orientation   Score   Total

What is the	day:	_____	1	
	date:	_____	1	
	month:	_____	1	
	year:	_____	1	
	season:	_____	1	_____ (5)
What is the	city:	_____	1	
	state:	_____	1	
	county:	_____	1	
	building:	_____	1	
	floor:	_____	1	_____ (5)

2. Registration

Name three objects and ask the patient to recall all three objects. (Give one point for each correct answer. Repeat until patient gets all three objects.) _____ (3)

3. Attention and Calculation

Serial 7's: Ask the patient to count subtract 7 from 100, and keep subtracting 7 from each answer. (Stop after 5 answers, score one point for each correct answer.) Alternate: Spell world backward. (Score one point for each correctly placed letter.) _____ (5)

4. Recall

After 2 minutes, ask for the 3 objects named in question 2. (Score one point for each correct answer.) _____ (3)

5. Language

Point to a pencil and a watch. Ask the patient to name each of them. (Score one point for each correct answer.) _____ (2)

Ask the patient to repeat the following phrase: "No if's ands, or buts." (Give one point for the correct answer) _____ (1)

Ask the patient to perform the following command: "Take this piece of paper in your right hand, fold it in half, and lay it on the table." (Score one point for each correct step.) _____ (3)

Ask the patient to read and carry out the following written command: "Close your eyes." (Score one for the correct response) _____ (1)

Ask the patient to write a sentence. It must contain a noun and a verb and make sense. Ignore spelling errors. (Score one point if correct.) _____ (1)

6. Visuospatial

Ask the patient to copy a drawing of two interlocking pentagrams. There must be five sides to each pentagram and four interlocking sides.

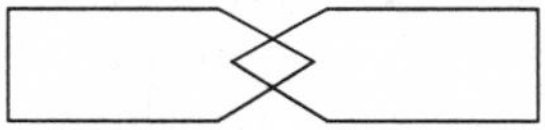

_____ (1)

Total _____ /30

FIGURE 8.1. Mini-Mental State Exam.

observing, often helps in obtaining information in the shortest amount of time. The symbols can be explained to the patient as the figure develops. Interestingly, information regarding family interactions is often volunteered when this method is used.

> An older man had finished describing his main problems. While the physician was diagramming his family, the patient admitted to having a brother whom he had not mentioned previously. His brother had died of a heart attack two years before. The patient expressed fear that his own high blood pressure might also lead to a heart attack. When asked how he dealt with his brother's death, he said, "Oh, I just put it out of my mind."

A family genogram will also provide a more accurate picture of marriage relationships and present support systems. It can serve as a method for both obtaining and recording a large amount of information, negating the need for a lengthy narrative account of the patient's family history. An example is shown in Figure 8.2.

Nutrition

Malnutrition is a common condition seen in old age. About one-third of those over 65 ingest inadequate nutrients.[15] Inadequate income, physical difficulties in preparing meals and shopping, inadequate knowledge of the nutritional shortcomings of high-carbohydrate "fast foods," and individual taste preferences all contribute to malnutrition. The patient should be queried as to what was eaten that day as a sample of daily intake. Asking how foods are bought and prepared may illuminate problems. Inquiries should be made into the use of home-delivered meal programs, such as Meals on Wheels, or of food stamps.

Exercise

A phrase often used in the care of the older person is, "Use it or lose it." This admonition applies to a great number of bodily functions, such as muscle strength, gait stability, and cardiovascular reserve. It also applies to cognitive functioning. Not only is exercise a vital way of maintaining

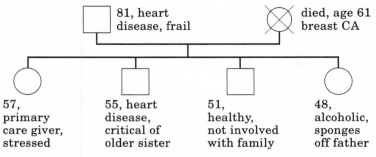

FIGURE 8.2. Family Genogram.

functions, but cessation of heretofore regular exercise can be a sign of physical illness or depression.

Regular exercise can take many forms in older people. Gardening, woodworking, performing lawn care, walking, and doing calisthenics are common and have been shown to promote fitness. These methods of maintaining physical function should be reinforced as a positive method of health promotion. Older patients should be informed that it is never too late to benefit from exercise as improvements in strength and functioning have been documented even in those who begin an exercise program in their nineties.[16]

Discussing Difficult Subjects

Two areas often neglected when interviewing an older person are sex and substance abuse. Contrary to popular belief, most men continue to be sexually active into their seventh or even eighth decades.[17] Although older women maintain sexual activity less frequently, this probably has more to do with lack of partners (women outnumber men almost two to one after the age of 75) than lack of interest. Indeed, over 65 percent of those over 65 expressed interest in sexual activities when interviewed.[18]

While it may not be mentioned in the first interview, sex should be discussed as the doctor-patient relationship develops. Some interviewers may have difficulty bringing up the subject, often because of preconceived notions about the image of someone who looks like their grandparent participating in sexual activities. The subject can be broached during the review of systems by asking, "Do you have any problems in your sexual life that you would like to discuss?"

Some older persons are at high risk for having substance abuse problems. Those with chronic illness, poverty, and depression are at highest risk. Many suffer from loneliness, a common source of problem drinking. Chronic pain syndromes can lead to narcotic abuse. Sleep disturbances are common in old age and may lead to excessive use of sedatives.

As with sexuality, it is perhaps difficult to conceive of a 75-year-old woman who reminds you of your grandmother being an alcoholic. Reticence in asking about alcohol intake is understandable but must be overcome if a complete history is to be taken. A simple question such as, "Have you ever had a problem with alcohol or medications?" will often begin the diagnostic interview. A formal set of screening questions such as the CAGE interview is also helpful (see Table 3.4).

PROBLEMS IN INTERVIEWING OLDER ADULTS

There are several common difficulties in interviewing older patients (Table 8.5). Some are a result of normal physiologic changes associated with aging, while others are due to illnesses. Both types of problems are discussed in this section.

Lack of a Specific Chief Complaint

Some older persons have a multitude of chronic health problems. The interplay between these problems is complex and often unpredictable.

TABLE 8.5. Problems in Interviewing Older Adults

1. Lack of a specific chief complaint
2. Altered presentations of illness
3. Acceptance of illness as a "normal" change of age
4. Fear of being institutionalized
5. Physical illness presents as psychological problem, and vice versa

Hence, the chief complaint is likely to be less illuminating than with younger patients. The patient may first present a long-standing problem, one felt to be most important by the patient's children, or even one that the patient feels may be most interesting to the doctor. By asking the patient, "Which problem is bothering you the most right now?" one can help determine a path of diagnosis and treatment.

Altered Presentations of Illness

As people get older, they often speak of health problems in nonspecific terms. This phenomenon has several causes. Normal changes of age, such as decreased pain sensation, decreased nerve conduction velocity, and decreased temperature responses, can contribute to an altered reporting of illness. Patients may experience the pain of diverticulosis of the colon as a dull ache in the belly, rather than severe abdominal discomfort. Those with early cognitive disorders may not recall that they have been feeling ill. Some older patients may exhibit only confusion with a serious infection, such as pneumonia or urinary tract infection. Due to the patient's advanced age, the health care provider may attribute the confusion to an underlying cognitive problem rather than a treatable condition.

Many of the common presentations of medical problems are nonspecific. The most common of these include "slowing down," either physically or mentally; weakness or tiredness; dizziness or falling; "rheumatism" (by which the patient may mean joint pain, bone pain, or muscle tenderness); anorexia or weight loss; and decreased libido. These problems may have their genesis in a remediable cause and deserve investigation.

ACCEPTANCE OF ILLNESS AS
A "NORMAL" CHANGE OF AGE

Many of the afflictions experienced by an older person may be mistakenly perceived as a normal part of aging. Loss of hearing, poor vision, shortness of breath, decreased exercise tolerance, sexual dysfunction, and even incontinence, though treatable, may be perceived by the patient as just another part of "getting old." Unfortunately, because they are subject to the same myths about old age, clinicians may contribute to this attitude.

A 70-year-old widowed man reported to his physician that he had been impotent for the last six months. This was particularly distressing because impotence had rarely occurred in his life and he had recently developed a relationship with a new companion. He was contemplating marriage but was frightened due to his change of sexual function. When he told his physician of these problems, the doctor said, "Well, we all have to get old some day." The patient was later seen by a different physician, who changed his anti-hypertensive medications, and the problem was resolved.

Fear of Being Institutionalized

Some elderly patients may be reticent about discussing their problems openly. They may appear suspicious or even paranoid. Among the greatest fears of older persons is that of being "put away" or institutionalized. In the patient's mind, it is a representative of the health care system—a doctor, social worker, or nurse—who is most likely to initiate placement in a long-term care setting. A clear statement to the patient that the goal of an intervention is to extend or ensure the patient's capacity to live independently (if that is indeed the case) may help to allay this fear.

Physical Illness Presents as Psychological Problem, and Vice Versa

Finally, there is another aspect of the presentation of illness that tends to distinguish older from younger patients, namely, physical illness that presents itself as a psychological problem or vice versa. An elderly person with an organic illness may have no physical complaints, for example, the patient with pneumonia who presents with agitation rather than cough and fever. The symptoms of certain cancers, such as those of pancreas and lung, may be preceded by as much as six months by the onset of a major depression. Certain endocrine problems, such as hypothyroidism, commonly present with depression or psychosis.

The person with a severe psychological problem, such as depression, may not report feelings of helplessness and loss of interest in activities, but may instead complain of multiple aches and pains. Even a severely depressed patient may not report feelings of hopelessness or loss of libido. Only the common physical signs of depression, such as lack of energy and weight loss, may be mentioned.

There are a number of approaches to this difficult problem. A new, serious decline in an older person's health or functioning should never be ascribed to "getting old" without adequately investigating the possibility of covert problems. An accurate history of the decline, a complete physical exam, and appropriate diagnostic tests will usually uncover hidden illnesses that are being expressed as psychological symptoms. Occasionally an older person requires a trial of antidepressant medication after such an evaluation. But take heart, even the most experienced clinician may have difficulty distinguishing depression from organic illness in older patients.

CONCLUSION

There are a number of special considerations when interviewing an older patient. Certain aspects of the process of the interview, such as paying attention to sensory deficits and the importance of reminiscence are particularly important. The content of the history may also differ from that of a younger person. The wide variety of backgrounds and experiences, the diversity of medical problems, and altered presentations of illness require from the clinician a blend of practiced interviewing skills and a warm, therapeutic approach.

REFERENCES

1. Adams, P. F., and G. Collins, "Measures of Health Among Older Persons Living in the Community." In *Health Statistics on Older Per-*

sons, United States, 1986, Vital and Health Statistics, Havlik, R. J., M. G. Liu, M. G. Kovar, et al. (eds.), Series 3, No. 25 DHHS Publ. No. (PHS) 87–1409. Public Health Service, Washington, D.C., U.S. Government Printing Office, June, 1987.

2. Von Leden, H., "Speech and Hearing Problems in the Geriatric Patient," *Journal of American Geriatric Society*, 25:422–426, 1977.

3. Harrigan, J. A., T. Heidotting, and K. Fox, "Analysis of Verbal Behavior Between Physicians and Geriatric Patients," *Family Practice Residents Journal*, 9:131–145, 1990.

4. Comstock, L. M., E. M. Hooper, J. M. Goodwin, and J. S. Goodwin, "Physical Behaviors that Correlate with Patient Satisfaction," *Journal of Medical Education*, 57:105–112, 1982.

5. Jones, T. V., and M. E. Williams, "Rethinking the Approach to Evaluating Mental Functioning of Older Persons: The Value of Careful Observations," *Journal of American Geriatric Society*, 36:1128–1134, 1988.

6. Kemp, B., "The Psychosocial Context of Geriatric Rehabilitation." In *Geriatric Rehabilitation*, Kemp, B., K. Brummel-Smith, and J. W. Ramsdell (eds.). Austin, TX: Pro-Ed Press, 1990. p. 53.

7. Brody, E., "Parent Care as a Normative Family Stress," *Gerontologist*, 25:19–29, 1985.

8. Sier, H. C., "Urinary Incontinence." In *Ambulatory Geriatric Medicine*, Yoshikawa, T. T., E. L. Cobbs and K. Brummel-Smith (eds.). St. Louis: Mosby Publications, 1993. p. 218.

9. Rubenstein, L. Z., "Falls." In *Ambulatory Geriatric Medicine*, Yoshikawa, T. T., E. L. Cobbs, and K. Brummel-Smith (eds.). St. Louis: Mosby Publications, 1993. p. 296.

10. Blazer, D., D. C. Hughes, and L. K. George, "The Epidemiology of Depression in an Elderly Community Population," *Gerontologist*, 27: 281–287, 1987.

11. Yesavage, J. A., T. L. Brink, T. L. Rose, et al., "Development and Validation of a Geriatric Depression Screening Scale: A Preliminary Report," *Journal of Psychiatric Research*, 17:37–49, 1983.

12. Mahoney, J., T. J. K. Drinka, R. Abler, et al., "Screening for Depression: Single Question Versus Geriatric Depression Scale," *Journal of American Geriatric Society*, 42:1006–1008, 1994.

13. Jones, T. V., and M. E. Williams, "Rethinking the Approach to Evaluating Mental Functioning of Older Persons: The Value of Careful

Observations," *Journal of American Geriatric Society*, 36:1128–1134, 1988.

14. Folstein, M. F., S. Folstein, and P. R. McHuth, "Mini-Mental State: A Practical Method for Grading the Cognitive State of Patients for the Clinician," *Journal of Psychiatric Research*, 12:189–193, 1975.

15. Beattie, B. L., and V. Y. Loiue, "Nutrition and Health in the Elderly." In *Clinical Aspects of Aging*, Reichel, W. (ed.). Baltimore: Williams & Wilkins, 1989. p. 213.

16. Fiaterone, M. A., E. C. Marks, N. D. Ryan, C. N. Meredith, L. A. Lipsitz, and W. J. Evans, "High-Intensity Strength Training in Nonagenarians: Effects on Skeletal Muscle," *Journal of American Medical Association*, 263:3029–3033, 1990.

17. McCarthy, P., "Geriatric Sexuality: Capacity, Interest and Opportunity," *Journal of Gerontological Nursing*, 5:20–24, 1979.

18. Pfeiffer, E., and G. Davis, "Determinants of Sexual Behavior in the Elderly," *Journal of American Geriatric Society*, 20:151–158, 1972.

9

CONTINUING CARE

KEY POINTS

1. Patients consult doctors because of a new medical problem, to discuss ongoing treatment plans, and to vent their feelings about psychosocial problems.
2. Patients have certain expectations from a visit to the doctor but seldom express them openly.
3. Listening for illness attributions is important.
4. Telling the patient what is wrong and what is to be done changes the interview style to physician-centered.
5. At the conclusion of the interview the patient may divulge hidden reasons for the visit.

This chapter focuses on interviewing as it relates to the continuing care of patients in the hospital, the office, or the clinic. Topics discussed are how to determine the reasons for the patient's visit, his expectations, his perception of the cause of the problem, opening and closing the interview, and informing the patient of the diagnosis and treatment.

REASONS FOR THE PRIMARY CARE VISIT

Patients consult doctors for many reasons. Some visits are for urgent problems and it is quite clear why the patient is there. Other patients with chronic diseases come for regularly scheduled appointments to monitor the disorder. In many instances, however, the physician wonders initially why the patient has come. The symptoms may be so minor that a visit to the doctor would seem unnecessary. It has been shown that many persons who are sick don't visit doctors at all while those who go to the doctor may be no more physically ill than those who don't.[1]

But there is always an important reason why the patient has decided to visit a doctor. In continuing care, it is often related to psychosocial distress.[2] Patients may visit physicians because of stress in their lives, feelings of social isolation, or simply to get information they believe the physician can provide. Patients with mental illness often use primary care physicians for psychiatric care if they do not have a mental health care provider or insurance that covers psychiatric visits. In such instances the patient may initially describe physical symptoms, and the real reason for coming will emerge only after careful interviewing.

During times of significant stress people often complain of a variety of physical and emotional symptoms. Headaches, stomachaches, nervousness, and irritability are a few examples. Most patients with stress-related symptoms sense that they are not mentally ill but need a doctor's reassurance that their reactions are not abnormal. They may also be in search of guidance about how to cope with the stress. Socially isolated persons often see physicians because they expect to be listened to and can feel some connection to another person. Indeed, for some elderly patients with disabilities, a physician may be their only means of having a social experience. Patients often see physicians to get information about communicable diseases, to order special medical equipment, or to learn more about the disease of a family member.

THE PATIENT'S EXPECTATIONS

It is important to understand what it is that the patient expects from going to the doctor. Kravitz and colleagues[3] defined patient expectations as those elements of care patients consider necessary for the physician to provide as part of a visit. Here are a few examples from clinical practice in the patients' own words.

- "I expect the doctor to listen, at least for the first five or six minutes."
- "I expect the doctor to define and clarify the problem, to name it."
- "I expect the doctor to discuss treatment or lack of treatment."
- "I expect the doctor to examine me and order some tests."
- "I expect to be given medicine to make me well."
- "When I make an appointment to go to a doctor's office, it is because something is wrong with me physically. I'm sick. I don't want the doctor to think I'm stupid or that there is nothing wrong, that I'm a woman who just imagines aches and pains to get attention. I have to justify myself why I am calling, why I go."
- "I expect the doctor to give me his undivided attention, not to be on the phone with other patients, no shuffling papers. I need to think he listens and hears me. It doesn't take long to get the feeling of attention. I, in turn, will listen the best I can. I may be in pain, exhausted, fearful, but I will do as the doctor suggests."
- "I don't expect to wait for more than 15 minutes every time I see the doctor."
- "I expect the doctor to ask me about all the medicines I'm taking."
- "I expect the doctor to ask me what I've already done to help myself."

As these responses indicate, it is difficult to be aware of the patient's expectations unless one asks. Patients are not likely to spontaneously make expectations known to the physician.

Mary Shelton, a 68-year-old clinical psychologist who had become severely anemic as a result of a bleeding, benign gastric ulcer, continued to complain of "not feeling well" for months after receiving blood transfusions and after the ulcer had healed. "Not feeling well" was her expression of a concern that something else might be wrong with her. She complained of a sense of fatigue she had not experienced before the bleeding ulcer. She realized that she was slightly depressed and at each visit described her difficulty in getting through her daily schedule of patients because of the fatigue. During one of these visits, the physician asked her what sort of expectations she had for that particular visit. To the surprise of the physician, she said, "I was aware of the beating of my heart when I was anemic. It got better after the transfusions but has now been back for several months. It bothers me particularly when I'm trying to get to sleep at night. I mentioned it to you several weeks ago but you didn't do anything about it. I really expected you to take it more seriously." The patient was then examined and found to have frequent extrasystoles that were responsible for her concern regarding her heart. She appeared relieved when further studies were advised.

In this instance, the physician might not have heard her tell him of her awareness of her heart because he may have assumed that the complaint was part of her anxiety and depression.

Learning about the patient's expectations may not be foremost in the mind of the primary care doctor, who is likely pressed to see one patient after another in a short period of time, listen to their symptoms, examine them, arrive at a diagnosis, and begin treatment. Yet eliciting the explicit expectations of the patient has been associated not only with increased patient satisfaction but also with symptom improvement and greater compliance.[4] There are several advantages to considering the patient's expectations. First, learning about them may further one's understanding of the clinical problems. A patient complaining of chest pain on exertion, angina, would probably expect the doctor to obtain an electrocardiogram, for example. Second, failing to address the patient's expectations may result in dissatisfaction with the care the patient receives.

In the study by Kravitz and colleagues,[3] patients were asked the following question before their visit to the doctor: "Realizing that it is not possible for your doctor to do everything in a single visit, please indicate the things you think are necessary for your doctor to do today." Twenty-eight elements of care, chosen by the doctors, including various aspects of the interview, the physical examination, laboratory tests, medication, counseling, and referral, were presented to the patients to identify their pre-visit expectations. Following the visits, the patients were asked to look again at the list and indicate whether or not the items identified on the list had been addressed. Finally, an overall visit satisfaction score was requested. The study showed that patients do have certain expectations, and that if their expectations are not met, they are less satisfied with their medical care. The nature of their illness, how they were likely to get better, and the results of blood tests were rated as very important by most of the volunteers. The study also showed that while patients have certain expectations, they might not voice them unless given the opportunity.

During the interview the clinician should include questions aimed at eliciting the patient's expectations. This is best accomplished when the clinician has been able to establish a climate in which the patient feels free to voice concerns. There are, however, certain groups of patients whose expectations are particularly important to determine. One group includes patients who have been described as "worried-well," those who do not present with easily identifiable illnesses and whose symptoms do not seem serious enough to warrant a visit to the physician. Another group consists of patients with different social and cultural backgrounds than the interviewer's. These patients are likely to have expectations that are foreign to the experience of the physician. With all such patients the clinician might say, "I think it would be helpful if you were to tell me what you expected would happen today as a result of this visit." When an open-ended question such as, "What kind of troubles are you having?" does not result in much information, a follow-up question such as, "How can I be of help to you?" might allow such patients to describe their expectations.

ILLNESS ATTRIBUTIONS

Illness attribution is the term used to describe the patients' beliefs about the cause of their illnesses. Most patients have such ideas. A mother might attribute her child's cold to getting his feet wet. The patient with an ulcer usually points to stress as a cause, though some will blame their diet. More serious illnesses such as heart attacks are often attributed to such causes as working too hard, not getting enough exercise, or being careless about diet. Those with strong Judeo-Christian religious beliefs may perceive the illness as punishment for their sins. Patients of other cultures may have beliefs that are very different than those of the interviewer.

It is valuable to learn about the patient's concerns or beliefs about what may be wrong. This may clarify the reason for the visit. A headache, for example, becomes more than a headache when a member of the family has recently been diagnosed as having a brain tumor. Illness attributions represent a window into the patient's psychosocial and cultural life. Patients frequently relate their symptoms to a particularly difficult situation at work or at home. Or the patient may describe the recent loss of a close friend and alert the physician to the problem of social isolation. Eliciting the patient's point of view involves him or her more fully as an active participant in the diagnostic process. This sense of being a partner in the process increases patient satisfaction.

In the course of an interview, patients may make some reference to what they believe has caused their illness, though often these beliefs are not stated openly and can be missed by the physician who is focusing on a pathophysiological explanation of the cause of the illness. It is also easy to dismiss notions that may seem unscientific to the physician. Listening carefully to the patient and keeping an open mind are keys to learning about illness attributions.

Patients are frequently more concerned about the feared cause of their symptoms than the symptoms themselves. For example, the appearance of an innocuous skin lesion may prompt the patient concerned about his HIV status to seek medical attention. The visit to the primary care physician should result not only in diagnosing and treating the lesion, but also in giving this patient license to talk about his sexual and other concerns. Limiting the discussion to the biomedical problems produces less patient satisfaction than if the psychological issues are also addressed.[5]

Attributions come from different sources. They may arise from the patient's own experiences with illness. For example, adolescents and young patients who have had infectious mononucleosis in the past often attribute any subsequent infection with symptoms of a sore throat and swollen glands to a recurrence of "mono." Adults who have previously had malaria often worry about its recurrence years later when they experience chills and fever from any cause.

A family history of serious or fatal illness is a common source of concern to first-degree relatives and may be reflected in their worries when they become ill. Children or siblings of those who have died of heart disease or cancer are likely to worry about any symptoms resembling those of their afflicted family members. Worry about Alzheimer's disease is common in middle-aged or older patients who have a family member with this disorder and who become concerned about their own memory.

Similarly, close contact with illness outside the family is likely to affect the perception of one's own symptoms. A heart attack striking a fellow worker will often cause associates of the same age to seek medical attention for any symptoms resembling those of the victim. Contact with illness by medical students, house staff, and even experienced physicians can cause them to worry that their minor symptoms are the result of serious or even fatal disease.

Patients' attributions can also derive from the social milieu in which they live. Illness is a common topic of discussion among family, friends, and even acquaintances. This is particularly the case with increasing age when comments about a person's health are likely to replace the usual social greetings. "You are looking well," is likely to replace, "It's good to see you again." Newspapers, magazines, radio, and television devote much space to medical topics. Widely publicized cases of disease in celebrities are likely to make others fear they may be suffering from the same disorder.

If a patient does not divulge his ideas about the cause of his symptoms, one should ask, "What do you think is the cause of your trouble?" especially when the patient hints at but doesn't come out with his concerns.

PATIENT: The cause of my trouble?

DOCTOR: You seem reluctant to tell me the cause. Perhaps you feel that I wouldn't believe you.

PATIENT: Well, my two best friends have the same disease I have, fever, swollen glands, and sweats.

DOCTOR: And?

PATIENT: Well, I think I have polymyalgia rheumatica, just like they have.

Such a question is also in order when the patient's symptoms are vague and don't fit a recognizable disease pattern or when the symptoms are minor but attended by unusual concern.

Patients with different cultural backgrounds may perceive and describe their symptoms in a manner quite foreign to the interviewer's experience. Their thoughts about what is wrong are shaped by the characteristic beliefs of their culture of origin. These patients may not talk about their illness attributions without encouragement from the physician for fear that they may appear foolish or uneducated. When they are helped to talk about them, however, the clinical picture will become clearer.

A 60-year-old Canadian-born wife of a professor of medieval history had finally died after six weeks of hospitalization following an unsuccessful cardiopulmonary resuscitation. The physician agreed to meet the Viennese-born husband at the mortuary the following morning to sign the death certificate. "When are you going to do the heart stab?" asked the husband. "The heart stab?" the physician asked. Then he learned for the first time of the wife's fear of waking up in the hearse, finding herself alive. The historian described a "heart stab" as a stab through the heart to make certain the patient is dead. It was his belief that this was commonly done in Vienna when he was growing up. After further discussion, the doctor convinced the husband that he was not going to do a "heart stab" and finally satisfied him by suggesting an embalming.

PREPARING TO SEE THE PATIENT

It is important to review the patient's records before seeing him. A hospitalized patient is usually seen by more than one physician. A patient with a complicated illness may be attended by several consultants in the course of a 24-hour period. Physicians on duty when the primary care doctor is off call may also visit the patient. Their progress notes and consultations should be reviewed before seeing the patient. In addition, many other health professionals are involved in the patient's care including nurses, physical and occupational therapists, respiratory therapists, speech therapists, and others. Their records often provide information that complements and may at times differ from that of the primary physician. Nurses, for example, have the most contact with the patient and often see him or her in a different light than the attending doctor, whose visit is likely to be more brief.

Some physicians carry the chart with them when they make rounds and thumb through the pages searching for laboratory results while talking with the patient. This behavior can be upsetting to patients who expect the physician to know what has been happening to them since the last hospital visit. The physician's visit is often the most important time of the day for a patient, who should be given his full attention.

Unlike the hospitalized patient whose immediate illness is the main issue, the ambulatory patient may have a long history of medical and surgical problems. Physicians must familiarize themselves with the past medical history before dealing with the present illness. This is best accomplished by referring to an updated problem and medication list and by quickly reviewing the progress note from the last visit. The few moments spent in reviewing the chart represent time well spent. The clinician will be better prepared for the present encounter, and the patient will be comforted to know that the physician is fully aware of the status of his or her problems.

Many managed care systems now use computerized medical records (CMR). The clinician can retrieve data to review the patient's past visits, current medications, the history of past medical problems and surgical procedures, laboratory reports, and even discharge summaries from the hospital. Some systems list past medications as well, along with a history of adverse drug reactions. This information is not only very helpful, it also prevents the physician from prescribing a drug with which the patient is known to have had problems.

Once the chart or CMR has been reviewed, the patient is ready to be seen. Ensuring privacy, if possible, is important. The nature of the greeting sets the tone for the meeting, then the interviewer is ready to begin the doctor-patient encounter.

OPENING THE CONTINUING CARE INTERVIEW

Greeting the Patient

As discussed in Chapter 2, addressing the patient by his proper title and surname is important. The patient may say, either during the introduction or as the interview progresses, that he would prefer being called by his first name. [6] Automatically calling patients by their first name, on the other hand, forces a level of intimacy or familiarity to which the patient has not consented. It also assigns to patients a lesser status since they are generally not expected to refer to physicians by their first names. Asking the patient how he would like to be addressed can produce an awkward moment since the patient may try to please the doctor by anticipating what he would like to hear.

Often the patient may have a name that is difficult to pronounce. In such cases, the patient will appreciate the clinician's effort to "get the name straight." If this is a new patient, it is equally important that the patient is told the student's or physician's name, and particularly the name of the physician in charge of his care.

In the ambulatory care setting, it is common practice for patients to be shown into an examining room by an aide or secretary. However, there are advantages to greeting the patient personally and showing him or her into the office or examining room. It is helpful to observe briefly patients' appearance and body posture as they wait to see the clinician. This can provide useful clues to their emotional and physical state.

At times, it is important to know whether the patient is alone or is accompanied by a relative or friend. Sometimes patients will request that the other person join them during the office or clinic visit. There is usually a good reason behind such a request. Some patients are quite anxious about their medical condition and feel supported by a family member or friend. Others are aware of impaired memory. Many family members worry that the patient cannot or will not tell the physician the whole story and want to be certain the patient is not failing to provide important information.

Ensuring Privacy

Pulling the curtain around the bed in a crowded hospital ward, emergency room, or clinic cubicle offers some sense of privacy to the patient. The close proximity of beds or cubicles to each other makes it difficult for a patient to talk about sensitive personal concerns. Patients who are on an open ward in the hospital are often not confined to their beds and can walk or be transported by wheelchair to a quieter and more private area nearby for the interview. The quality of the interview is immensely enhanced by attention to this important detail. When possible, the interview should take place either in the clinician's office or in a private room. A sense of privacy is also fostered by the behavior of the interviewer. Sitting close to the patient and establishing good eye contact are helpful. Good eye contact is best established when the patient and clinician are seated at the same level. Raising the head of the patient's bed helps. On the other hand, standing above the patient not only discourages a feeling of privacy but can be intimidating.

Beginning with a Comment or an Open-Ended Question?

Students in their clerkship, house staff, and physicians in practice see their hospitalized patients daily, and each time they are faced with the same issue of how to open the interview. The patient's appearance and behavior often dictates whether the clinician comments on his or her medical or emotional state. "Your breathing seems a lot easier this morning, Mrs. Rafferty," would be an appropriate reaction to a patient who had been hospitalized with severe shortness of breath and is now much improved. To a woman who is no longer experiencing pain, one could comment on how much more comfortable she appears. Most patients' nonverbal behavior will reveal how they are handling their hospitalization. Depression is common and will be evidenced by the facial appearance and voice. "You look a little sad this morning," will encourage the patient to talk about her concerns, feelings of isolation from family and friends, or reaction to the nature or progress of her illness. On the other hand, if no clues to the patient's physical or emotional state are given, one might open with a remark such as, "Well, Mr. Smythe, how is it going today?" This type of opening question allows Mr. Smythe to talk about his illness or concerns.

The opening exchange between the clinician and patient in the outpatient setting depends on the nature of the visit. Is the patient returning to the clinic after a recent hospitalization? Does the patient have a chronic problem that requires regular periodic visits? Or is this a new patient with problems not familiar to the clinician?

Patients returning to the clinic after a hospitalization will be asked about their progress since their recent discharge. "How have you been feeling since you left the hospital?" is preferable to immediately asking specific questions relating to the recent illness. A patient's main problem at home may be psychosocial or economic, and the open-ended question allows him to talk about these aspects of his life in contrast to the physician-centered approach, which may limit the interview to physical symptoms.

In seeing patients with long-standing chronic illnesses or new patients with illnesses yet to be diagnosed, the same principles of open-ended, patient-centered interviewing should be followed. The patient with a chronic illness returning for a regularly scheduled appointment may have new concerns, as in the following example:

An 86-year-old widow came to the physician's office for a regular appointment to have her blood pressure checked. In response to the question, "How have things been going for you since I last saw you?" she said, "I'm terribly depressed." She had seen an ophthalmologist a month earlier who had told her that she needed cataract surgery and that she also had glaucoma. "And this has made you depressed?" the physician responded. "Yes, but I'm too old to have surgery. Besides, I can't put the drops into my right eye without my daughter's help," she said and went on to tell the story of her foster father who, as a child, had received the wrong medicine in his eye and had gone blind. "Since I was a child I've been afraid of going blind," she added.

This patient had been treated over the years for many medical problems, including osteoarthritis, esophagitis with a stricture requiring dilatation, a total knee replacement, and hypertension. In all that time the physician had not learned of her fear of blindness. He might have been tempted to begin the interview by inquiring about the status of one or more of her physical problems. Such an opening, however, would not have given her the same opportunity to talk about her concern that she might go blind.

"Tell me what sort of troubles you are having?" or some variation of this open-ended question is the best way to begin an interview with a new patient. But patients may not feel free on the first visit to talk about the more personal issues that accompany their medical illness.

A 46-year-old married woman was seen by her doctor because of severe, recurrent headaches. On returning to her physician after the initial office visit, she was asked, "How are things going for you?" She began to talk about how much she loved working in the bookstore at the university where she was employed as a cashier. She mentioned that she enjoyed the people in the store and how nice they were to her. "It's so different from the way my husband treats me," she said. She went on to talk about how critical he was of her gain in weight, and how tired he was of her complaining about her headaches. Subsequent visits began in the same way. Gradually her life was revealed to the physician. This might not have occurred if the visits had begun with questions directed to her headaches.

There are many patients whose appearance or behavior is so striking that the clinician may decide to comment on it rather than begin with an open-ended question. For example, a patient with an acute attack of gout involving the foot will be in obvious pain and will limp as he enters the office. "You look like you are in a lot of pain, Mr. Woodworthy," would be an appropriate remark. Similarly, if the patient appears sad or anxious, a comment about this would be in order.

Patients well known to the physician appreciate a reference to a personal event discussed during the last visit. A quick perusal of the chart before the patient is seen will remind the physician of the event.

ALLOTTING TIME

Nelson and McLemore[7] have reported that the average primary care visit in the United States is less than 20 minutes: about 14 minutes for family practitioners and 19 for internists. Of course, some visits may be for only a few minutes while others may be considerably longer than 20 minutes. In managed care environments, there may even be less time for the visit. When time is limited, it is important that the clinician use the available time wisely. Roter and Hall[8] have shown that half the time allotted to the patient's visit is consumed by the physician's reading the notes of the previous visit and interruptions by telephone calls from other patients, doctors and agencies, or pharmacies. Time is also spent writing chart notes and prescriptions.

Giving the patient undivided attention can overcome some of the difficulties imposed by the limitations of time. Attentiveness is enhanced when the clinician establishes good eye contact and conveys a sense of being unhurried. In such instances, the patient may report that the physician behaved as though he had only one patient and was prepared to spend as much time as was necessary.

Audiotapes by Korsch and colleagues[9] of visits to a pediatric clinic confirm that what one does with the time available is the most important consideration. Some patients complained of not having time to tell the doctor their story when in reality the interview had lasted 30 to 40 minutes. A review of the tapes showed that most of the physician's time had been spent asking questions and verbally sparring with the mothers of pediatric patients.

After a few minutes, the experienced clinician knows whether the patient's problems can be sorted out within the time allotted for the visit or will require more time than has been scheduled. Those patients needing more time than anticipated can be satisfied by focusing attention on the present illness and then making a follow-up appointment to explore the problems more fully. Obviously, patients with urgent problems need immediate attention.

In the practice of primary care medicine, some patients will come with a whole range of problems that cannot be fully addressed in a 20 to 30 minute visit:

> The patient, a 78-year-old man, had recently moved to the community from another state. He was somewhat apologetic as he summarized his extensive medical history, which included two cardiac by-pass operations, repair of an abdominal aneurysm, a history of bladder cancer with resection and radiation, carcinoma of the prostate, and a swollen leg. It was agreed that with the exception of the swelling of his right leg, follow-up of the other problems could wait a few days until his medical records arrived from his previous physician. The patient accepted this, and the medical visit was limited to the problems with his leg.

Occasionally, a patient will be seen with a long list of problems, none of which are really urgent or life-threatening. Quill suggests asking the patient what he wants to focus on in the time available and scheduling another appointment to discuss the other problems.[10]

INFORMING THE PATIENT WHAT IS WRONG AND WHAT IS TO BE DONE

This aspect of the primary care visit is sometimes called the exposition phase, a time when the physician informs the patient of the diagnosis and proposed management of the illness. It is a time when the clinician switches gears from being patient-centered to physician-centered as he or she describes the diagnosis and treatment plan to the patient. It usually occurs after the examination has been completed. Often the diagnosis is obvious after the physical examination, and the patient can be told what is wrong and what the course of treatment should be. When the clinician cannot make the diagnosis before laboratory or other studies are done, he or she will have to present the findings to date and the reasons for wanting further studies. In either case, this phase of doctor-patient communication is often more difficult than the data-gathering phase that preceded it. Much of the difficulty is due to clinicians' tendency to use technical language. Physicians who use their accustomed technical language generally act as though their patients understand them, and patients generally act as if they understand. In one study patients told the doctor they did not understand only 15 percent of the time when an unfamiliar term was used.[11]

A 62-year-old man was forced to stop jogging one day along the beach by crushing chest pain. He rested for five minutes until the pain began to subside. He did not tell the nearby lifeguards of his distress but decided to walk home slowly. The pain persisted for about an hour. By the next morning, he was feeling better but was worried about what had happened to him while jogging. He consulted his primary care physician. An electrocardiogram showed that he had had a heart attack. When the physician encountered disbelief and resistance to being transported next door to the hospital, a cardiologist was brought into the office. She explained the situation to the patient: "Your electrocardiogram shows you have had an anterior myocardial infarction. You need to have serial enzymes, and your EKG monitored. Then we'll probably have to do an angiogram on you in the morning." The patient, who had said nothing during the cardiologist's exposition, then asked, "Does this mean I have to go to the hospital?" He had not understood a word of her jargon.

Physicians may even thoughtlessly use medical terms when they don't expect the patient to understand. Since doctors devote so much of the primary care visit to discussing the diagnosis and treatment recommendations, it is important that the time be spent fostering better communication.

Another problem is the frequent discrepancy between what patients want to know and what physicians think they would like to know. While patients put the highest priority on the diagnosis, prognosis, and origin of their conditions, physicians consistently underestimated their patients' desire for information in these areas. Instead, they thought patients were more interested in discussing treatment issues.[12] This explains why so many clinic patients interviewed have little idea about the nature of their illness, its name, what caused it, or what is to be expected as a result of treatment.

Golden and colleagues[13] suggested guidelines for providing information to patients. Assure that rapport has been established and that the patient is able to give his full attention to the physician (i.e., is not getting dressed, not trying to discuss another subject). When explaining a medical condition, its treatment and its expected outcome, use words the patient understands (Table 9.1).

Here is an example of clear communication:

"Mr. Jones, I would like to talk with you about what is wrong with you, the tests we will need to do, the medicine you will need to take, what you can do for yourself and how I think you will get along. What is wrong is that you have high blood pressure, which is often called hypertension. We really don't know what causes it, but we are going to do a few tests to see if it is affecting your system in any way. You are not really having any trouble now. As you know, the nurse found your blood pressure to be high at work or you might not even have known about it. I don't expect it is going to give you any trouble as long as you always remember to take the medicine I'm going to prescribe. I don't want you to let the medicine run out because it is important that we keep your blood pressure normal to prevent complications. Since you are feeling perfectly well, you might be tempted to stop taking the medicine at some point, but you can't afford to let the blood pressure go up, as it will if you stop treatment. Now, you can help yourself by losing weight, and we will talk about how you can do that. You can also check your own blood pressure at home and keep a record for me. I'm going to explain how you can get a machine to check your own blood pressure. Then we will set you up for another appointment in about a month to see how it's all going."

In this example, it would also be helpful to ask the patient to tell you what he has understood from the discussion. Some of the explanation may need to be repeated; written information is helpful in this regard. Enlisting the help of a family member would be important in following a program of dietary restriction as well as providing patient support. By paying attention to all of these issues in explaining the diagnosis and treatment, one increases the likelihood of compliance with the therapeutic process.

TABLE 9.1. Guidelines for Providing Information to Patients

1. Establish rapport.
2. Ensure patient gives full attention to discussion.
3. Use words the patient understands.
4. Summarize.

INFORMED CONSENT

All patients deserve to be given adequate information about their problem and its recommended treatment so that they can make an informed decision. While much of the discussion about "informed consent" has centered on the legal aspects of documenting that the patient has had a procedure explained and understands the risks, the real issue in informed consent is whether the patient has received enough information to make an educated decision. Informed consent is conceived of having four components: (1) that the treatment or Procedure is explained in terms the patient can understand; (2) Alternative treatments, as well as what is likely to occur if no treatment is given, are discussed; (3) the Risks of the treatment are discussed; and (4) the patient is given the opportunity to ask Questions (Table 9.2). Each patient will have a different need for information and explanation. The clinician who approaches this process in a patient-centered manner is more likely to have a patient who truly understands the nature of the decision and the risks involved. Insurance companies have found that physicians who communicate the process of informed consent well are much less likely to be sued, even if a bad outcome occurs.

CLOSURE

Closure refers to the process of ending the medical visit. It is an important time in the doctor-patient interaction. What happens during this period may affect the patient's satisfaction with the medical care given as well as his or her compliance with the physician's recommendations.

TABLE 9.2. Components of Informed Consent

P	procedure
A	alternatives
R	risks
Q	questions

A good interview will include a smooth transition between the exposition phase and closure. There should be a short summary of the visit, a final check of the patient's understanding of the treatment plan, and consolidation of rapport.[14] "Well, I'd like you to call me in a few days if your sore throat or fever have not improved," might be such a transition statement as the physician initiates closure by beginning to rise from his chair, giving a signal to the patient that the visit is coming to a close.

Barsky has shown that patients' hidden agendas may surface in the closing moments of the visit.[1] He suggests that these late disclosures of medical or psychosocial concerns occur because they have not been addressed earlier, either during the body of the interview or during the exposition phase. But there may be other reasons. Sometimes patients are afraid to deal with certain issues and wait until the end of the visit when they know there is no more time to spend with the physician. The physician's invitation, "In closing, is there anything else you would like to mention?" provides them with one last chance to talk about the real reason for the visit. For some patients it may take the entire visit to develop the necessary confidence and trust in their doctor.

Closure is a time when the interview is more physician-centered and a time to make certain that the patient understands the problem and treatment. It is also the time to schedule a return appointment if indicated, or to advise the patient to phone back to report on the status of the illness, or for the doctor to convey the results of laboratory tests. Finally, at the close of the visit an expression of the physician's appropriate concern and encouragement can help foster a strong relationship that is important to continuing care.

REFERENCES

1. Barsky, A. J., "Hidden Reasons Some Patients Visit Doctors," *Annals of Internal Medicine*, 94:492–498, 1981.
2. Suchman, A. L. and D. A. Mathews, "What Makes the Patient-Doctor Relationship Therapeutic? Exploring the Connexional Dimension of Medical Care," *Annals of Internal Medicine*, 108:125–130, 1988.
3. Kravitz, R. L., D. W. Cope, and V. Bhrany, "Internal Medicine Patients' Expectations for Care," *Journal of General Internal Medicine*, 9:75–81, 1994.
4. Eraker, S. A., J. P. Kirscht, and M. H. Becker, "Understanding and Improving Patient Compliance," *Annals of Internal Medicine*, 100:258–268, 1984.
5. Uhlman, R. F., W. B. Carter, and T. S. Inue, "Fulfillment of Patient Requests in a General Medicine Clinic," *American Journal of Public Health*, 74:257–258, 1984.
6. Lazare, A., "Shame and Humiliation in the Medical Encounter," *Archives of Internal Medicine*, 147:1653–1658, 1987.
7. Nelson, C., and T. McLemore, National Center for Health Statistics, *The National Ambulatory Medical Care Survey: U.S. 1975–1981*, and 1985 trends. Washington, D.C.: U.S. Government Printing Office.
8. Roter, D. L., and J. A. Hall, *Doctors Talking with Patients*. Westport, Connecticut: Auburn House, 1992. p. 87.
9. Korsch, B. M., E. K. Gozzi, and V. Francis, "Gaps in Doctor-Patient Communication," *Pediatrics*, 42:855–871, 1968.
10. Quill, T. E. "Partnerships in Patient Care: A Contractual Approach," *Annals of Internal Medicine*, 98:228–234, 1983.
11. McKinlay, J. B. "Who is Really Ignorant—Physician or Patient?" *Journal of Health and Social Behavior*, 16:3–11, 1975.
12. Kindelan, K., and G. Kent, "Concordance Between Patients' Information Preferences and General Practitioners' Perceptions," *Psychology and Health*, 16:399–409, 1987.
13. Golden, A., M. Grayson, E. Bartlett, et al., "The Doctor-Patient Relationship: Communication and Patient Education." In *Principles of Ambulatory Medicine*, J. N. Gardner, (ed.). Baltimore: Williams and Wilkins, 1986. pp. 30–40.
14. White, J., W. Levinson, and D. Roter, "The Closing Moments of the Medical Visit," *Journal of General Internal Medicine*, 9:24–28, 1994.

10

GIVING BAD NEWS AND DISCUSSING ADVANCE DIRECTIVES

Geoffrey H. Gordon, M.D.

KEY POINTS

1. Giving bad news requires skill and tact; both can be learned.
2. There is always room for hope in the face of a life-threatening illness.
3. The physician can help the patient plan for the future.
4. The physician should bring up the subject of advance directives.
5. When talking with patients about bad news or advance directives, be aware of your own feelings.

This chapter is divided into two sections. Each one addresses a communication dilemma commonly faced by physicians but rarely discussed in medical school or residency training. The first section deals with giving bad news to patients and families, and the second deals with discussing advance directives. In each section, the goals are to review pertinent background material, identify some common barriers to communication, suggest techniques to facilitate effective communication, and discuss some common problem areas.

GIVING BAD NEWS

Background

The goal of this section is to review some common issues in giving bad news. The focus is on the physician's role in giving the diagnosis of cancer, although the general principles apply to a variety of "bad news" situations. Despite these suggestions, there is rarely a single "right way" to give bad news, and it is never easy.

Physicians in other eras and cultures have traditionally avoided giving patients bad news. In the United States, however, the percentage of physicians who tell cancer patients the diagnosis has risen from 3 to 10 percent to over 94 percent in the last three decades.[1] This increase represents desire for greater patient autonomy and self-determination, greater public awareness of advances in cancer diagnosis and treatment, and greater scrutiny of the physician-patient relationship by administrative and allied health professionals. Research into the doctor-patient relationship has also shown that giving patients information can reduce their isolation and fear and help them mobilize their resources and coping skills. Surveys of cancer patients over the last three decades suggest that physicians have always underestimated the patients' desire to be told if they have cancer.[2]

Patients' Barriers to Communication

Some patients have more than the usual reluctance to hear, accept, and work with bad news. They may simply deny the reality of the news and angrily refuse to accept diagnostic or treatment recommendations. Alternatively, they may passively "give up" and rapidly lose function, or seek unrealistic cure through aggressive lifestyle changes. Bad news, like illness, tends to accentuate patients' usual coping styles, only some of which may promote healthy behaviors. Rather than change patients' characteristic coping styles, the task of the primary care physician is to strengthen healthy and adaptive defenses and to minimize damage from unhealthy ones.

Despite the devastating effect of bad news on patients' lives, studies suggest that patients can separate the "message" from the "messenger." For example, the way that parents are told that their child has a developmental disability or mental retardation affects the emotional state and attitude of both child and parents. A third to a half of parents in these studies were dissatisfied with how the news was given.[3,4]

Mrs. A. had worried about a lump in her neck for weeks. She tried not to think about her mother's long and futile battle with breast cancer. When her own lump hadn't gone away on its own, Dr. H. had wanted a biopsy. She felt that was fine, but wondered why he wanted her to be in the hospital? The lump was down near her collarbone; maybe that had something to do with it. Maybe it was too close to the heart.

The next morning, Dr. H. came into her room surrounded by a group of young doctors. He leaned against the wall and smiled down at Mrs. A. "Well, I have some good news and some bad news for you today. That lump in your neck is a kind of cancer called lymphoma. The good news is that when it responds to treatment, it responds better than the more benign types. The bad news is that it is less likely to respond. We'll know more about it later, after we run some more tests. In the meantime I want you to stay here so we can find out how far it's spread."

He turned to the students. "This is a 68-year-old woman who presented with a persistent left supraclavicular node and moderately severe anemia. Her biopsy shows a high-grade non-Hodgkin's lymphoma, what we used to call a diffuse histiocytic. She probably has bone marrow involvement. Let's go down to pathology and review her slides." He turned back to Mrs. A. "We'll come back and talk to you some more later on."

The doctors turned away and left the room. Mrs. A. pulled the covers up to her neck and stared out the window. She had never felt so alone and frightened in her life.

Barriers to Communication for Physicians

Physicians from ancient Greece to the recent past have avoided giving bad news, fearing effects more harmful than the diseases themselves. Perhaps they recognized the importance of faith and optimism in coping with disease, or perhaps they thought that giving bad news spoke poorly to their skills as practitioners. In medieval times, physicians were sometimes encouraged to be optimistic with patients but pessimistic with families. In this way credit could be taken either for miraculous healing powers, or for remarkable foresight, depending on whether the patient recovered or died.

Until recently, medical trainees learned how to give bad news by trial and error, doing it alone or with the advice of another trainee. Few physicians in training have seen experienced clinicians give bad news, although some have witnessed the task being passed on to a house officer, nurse, or even a family member. With the advent of communication skills training in medical schools and residency training programs, most physicians have now had some exposure to the knowledge, skills, and attitudes basic to giving bad news. Ethical and legal precedents now exist that oblige physicians to fully inform patients of their conditions and possible treatments.

Techniques for Giving Bad News

Considerations in giving bad news include preparation, choosing a setting, giving the news, providing emotional support, giving information, and closing the interview [5] (Table 10.1).

Preparing patients for the possibility of cancer can be done early in the workup. ("Mr. Jones, that shadow on your chest X-ray worries me. It could be an old scar, a little fluid, or even a cancer. I think we should do some more tests to find out exactly what it is.") Ask the patients how they would like to receive test results. ("Whatever the biopsy shows, I'm sure we have plenty to talk about—is there someone you'd like to come with you to that visit?") Also, be sure to coordinate your plans with others on the health care team, including consulting physicians who may learn and communicate the diagnosis to the patient or record it on the chart without your knowledge.

Bad news should always be given in person, by the physician. An exception is the patient who asks, "Is it cancer?" over the phone, in which case its best not to lie. Try to locate a private place to talk, and sit down with the patient to demonstrate your full attention and concern.

In giving the news, the most important step is assessing what the patient is ready to hear. Review or ask patients about what tests have

TABLE 10.1. Techniques for Giving Bad News

1.	Prepare the patient for the news
2.	Choose an appropriate setting
3.	Assess readiness to hear the news
4.	Give the news
5.	Provide emotional support
6.	Answer patient questions
7.	Close the interview
8.	Work with other team members
9.	Be aware of your own feelings

been done to date, what results mean to them, and what they are most concerned about. Some patients will immediately ask if it's cancer. Others will skirt the issue verbally or give nonverbal signals of discomfort. In this case, two methods can be used to slow down the message. One method is graded exposure. ("I'm afraid I have some bad news for you. This is more serious than we thought. There was some cancer in the biopsy.") The danger of this approach is that the physician may fail to finish with a clear, unambiguous statement that the patient has cancer. A second method is based on the observation that patients remember little of what is said to them after the diagnosis is given. In this method a most important message is presented first. ("Whatever I tell you in a moment, I want you to remember, the situation is serious, but there's plenty we can do. We'll have to work closely over the next several months.") This can be followed with "The biopsy shows that it's definitely cancer."

Receiving the diagnosis of cancer is still primarily an emotional rather than a cognitive event, and parients remember the physician's manner and attitude more vividly than technical details. For strong emotional reactions, the greatest challenge for physicians is to remain with patients and tolerate their distress. There are no "right things to say;" Dame Cicely Saunders, originator of the hospice movement in the United Kingdom, said, "The real secret is not what you tell your patients, but what you let your patients tell you."

Two common immediate emotional reactions are fear and grief.

Some patients experience and express these feelings as anger, which they may direct toward the physicians. ("I've always felt fine and followed your advice—there's got to be some mistake!" or, "Why didn't you find this sooner?") Rather than becoming defensive, acknowledge that many patients feel shortchanged and angry. Emphasize that the disease, not the doctor, is the enemy and that you will work together to fight it. For patients expressing grief, empathy statements can be useful. ("I can see this is a terrible blow for you, and that you're doing your best to cope. I want you to know that I'll continue to be your doctor and work with you on this.") A touch on the hand or shoulder is often supportive and reassuring. Finally, some patients will seem stunned or numb and will show little emotion. They may have others (for example, a close friend or minister) with whom they grieve. You can acknowledge their reaction and legitimize future expressions of feelings. ("I know this must be hard to believe or even think about. You may have some feelings later that you'd like to talk with me about. I'm always ready to listen.")

In addition to coping with feelings, most patients will want and need information about their disease. Cancer patients often want to know if they really have cancer, if it has spread, whether or not it is treatable and curable, and what treatment is like. Some patients want to know if and when they are going to die. Even with careful explanations, many patients have trouble assimilating much information at the time the bad news is given. Effective strategies in giving information are outlined in Table 10.2 and include using simple, clear words rather than medical jargon; giving small, digestible "chunks" of information at a time, checking patients' understanding of what has been said so far; and using

TABLE 10.2. Information-Giving Strategies

1.	Find out what patients already know
2.	Tailor information to "fill in the gaps"
3.	Use simple, clear words, pictures, or lists
4.	Avoid technical terms and medical jargon
5.	Give small amounts of information at a time
6.	Summarize and check patient's understanding
7.	Use handouts and other resources

handouts or other resources for patients to take home and read. One should answer tough questions directly and honestly. ("Yes, we are all going to die, but I don't know that you will die because of this cancer. There are statistics on how long people with your condition live, with and without treatment. But they are just averages. I can't predict how long you have.") Some physicians make audiotapes of bad news visits for patients to listen to more than once; 77 percent of 41 patients in one survey found this useful.[6] Some patients learn and gain emotional support from other patients with the same condition.

The most effective way to reach closure for the bad news visit is to provide an immediate plan of action for the future. Closure includes asking patients who else needs to know the news and if they would like help in conveying it. Patients will often see consultants and have more diagnostic testing, but will benefit from learning that you will still be their doctor. Some physicians like to prescribe a short course of medication for sleep or anxiety, but patients should be told that it is normal to be upset or to have trouble sleeping after receiving bad news. Finally, patients should be encouraged to write down questions that occur to them and bring them to the next visit.

A few additional considerations apply in death notification, or giving the bad news of the death of a loved one th a surviving family member. This is most difficult in unexpected, traumatic deaths. If the survivor is away from the hospital and must be notified by telephone, encourage him or her to come to the hospital prior to actual death notification, unless the survivor specifically asks about death. Once given the news, survivors will often want to see the deceased's body. This is an important part of the grieving process and should not be discouraged. Survivors tend to be most concerned about whether or not their loved one suffered or was alone at the time of death, and if there was anything they could have done to prevent it. Finally, survivors should be asked about anatomical gifts such as corneas, skin, or bone. Depending on the cause of death and comorbid conditions, the deceased may be eligible for organ donation. Many families find comfort in making an anatomical gift. Permission for autopsy can also be requested at this time. Many hospitals have policies and specially trained personnel who can follow up on these details once the issue is brought up by the notifying physician.

> Mr. Malone, a healthy 50-year-old, collapsed suddenly and unexpectedly at home. Paramedics found him to be in ventricular fibrillation. Resuscitation efforts en route to the hospital were unsuccessful and he was pronounced dead on arrival.
>
> The emergency room physician on call found Mrs. Malone in the waiting room and guided her to an empty office. He explained that, despite their best efforts, they could not save her husband. He sat with her for a few minutes as she wept and then asked if she wanted to view his body. At the bedside she said she didn't know what she should do next. The physician asked if her husband ever discussed funeral arrangements with her and explained that the hospital would arrange to have his body taken to the funeral home.
>
> He then asked if she and Mr. Malone had ever discussed organ donation. He explained that patients and families often take comfort in knowing that anatomical gifts of the skin, bone, or corneas will help another person get well. He mentioned that harvesting these organs would not disfigure Mr. Malone's body for an open-casket funeral, but that certain organs such as corneas needed to be taken soon. He then said he would ask the hospital's organ procurement specialist to contact her to answer her questions. He also suggested that she look carefully at her husband's driver's license, since many of them have a box to check if organ donation is desired.

Although it is still the physician's role to deliver the bad news, other health care professionals play important roles. Nurses in inpatient and outpatient settings can help witness and interpret the bad news for patients, help them verbalize their feelings and questions, and provide emotional support. Nurses are trained to assess patients' emotional and physical responses to treatment, their level of comfort and activity, and their expressed goals and progress toward these goals. Nurses who work with critically or terminally ill patients are often skilled at clarifying the overall direction and goals of care, and ensuring that treatment decisions are congruent with those directions and goals. Social workers are skilled at identifying resources, enhancing coping skills, and working with families. Chaplains can also assist in identifying and meeting patients' spiritual needs.

For physicians who give bad news, "taking your own pulse" is an invaluable skill. Physicians may need to identify and talk about their own grief with a trusted colleague before giving bad news to patients whom they have known for years. Physicians may worry that acknowledging or expressing feelings is "unprofessional" in the eyes of patients and colleagues; however, the reverse is often true. ("I know that doctor really cared for Jimmy when he shed a tear at the meeting.") Self-awareness and self-scrutiny can help physicians remain conscious of how their feelings and biases can affect treatment decisions. This also helps to avoid emotional burnout.

Problem Areas in Giving Bad News

Patients, families, and physicians are always fearful of losing hope. Many physicians have never learned how to foster hope and provide reassurance along with bad news. To physicians, hope often translates to cure, remission, or at least a treatment response. To patients, however, hope is often directed at a "moving target" that may begin with the possibility of cure, move to a goal of living until a next birthday or child's graduation, extend to living a life without pain, and finally be directed at dying peacefully at home, surrounded by loved ones. Hope and reassurance can be provided at the time of giving bad news in a variety of ways.[7,8] For example, consider using positive words (think of the difference between, "Your scan is negative," and, "Your scan shows that your liver is normal and healthy"). You can also present illness as a challenge. Most patients will have faced other illnesses or challenges and found new coping skills, as have patients with similar cancers ("I'm always surprised at how well patients do with . . ."). Finally, help patients understand that their thoughts, attitudes, and activities affect how their bodies feel. Teach the importance of learning to relax and to find new sources of pleasure and self-esteem. Warn patients about the danger of feeling that they have not done a good job of "being positive" if their disease progresses. Some patients will consistently fight the disease with a positive focus until the end, whereas others need permission to acknowledge and grieve their losses. Improved quality of life can never be guaranteed, but it remains the goal of these approaches.

Some patients specifically request not to be told bad news. They may harbor misconceptions about the disease or its treatment, and may even consider suicide if they were to receive certain kinds of news. Ask patients what the news would mean to them, or what they fear might happen, if they were to receive bad news. Explain the rationale for their knowing the news. ("Your job is to create the best environment for our medicines and treatments to work. This includes working with us to plan treatment, finding what parts of you are healthy and strong, and what areas still need some work. Your attitude and interest will affect how you feel.") If family members ask that patients not be given bad news, reassure them that unwanted information won't be forced on the patient. However, they should be told the rationale for the patient's knowing the news, as outlined above. Some families have had prior experiences with bad news, or strong cultural beliefs may underlie their wishes not to tell the patient. It may help to share your dilemma with the patient. ("Your family has told me that you'd prefer not to be informed about some important aspects of your care. What are your thoughts about this?")

Some patients are unable or unwilling to accept bad news such as a diagnosis of cancer. This is particularly frustrating when early treatment is potentially curative. Logical arguments and dire predictions aimed at persuading or convincing patients to accept treatment are rarely successful. Instead, try to respect denial as a generally useful, but currently maladaptive, coping mechanism. Explain that patients are often of "two minds." ("Many patients find this kind of diagnosis hard to believe. I can see that part of you wants to look on the bright side and stay hopeful. I wonder if you don't also have times when you wonder if this condition will stay or worsen. Let's talk about what we should do if that happens.") Expect to see day-to-day variation in what the patient believes and expects about the illness, and offer to answer any questions the patient might have. Document your conversations in the patient's chart to notify others on the health care team about the patient's reaction to the news; otherwise you may be blamed for not sharing bad news when in fact the patient is ambivalent about acknowledging it. Sometimes anticipating future needs makes the diagnosis more real for patients. ("Let's see how you're set up if your condition worsens. What kinds of decisions and plans should we try to make now, in case you're not feeling well enough to handle them in the future?")

DISCUSSING ADVANCE DIRECTIVES

Background

Patients have the ethical and legal right to refuse medical care, including life-sustaining treatment. When patients become too ill to make their own wishes known, the presumption is that they would want everything possible done to sustain life. However, this presumption has been increasingly challenged in clinical practice, survey-based research, and a series of dramatic court cases. Patients are now encouraged to plan for future illness or incapacity and to communicate these plans, preferably in writing, to their families and physicians. These "advance directives" can be oral or written, and general or specific. Written advance directives are now legal in most states and take the form either of a "living will" or a directive to physicians, or a durable power of attorney for health care in which patients appoint a spokesperson for health care decisions. Advance directives are only applicable when patients are unable to speak for themselves and are designed to direct (not necessarily limit) their medical care.

Patient preferences in advance of illness are stable 70 to 80 percent of the time.[9] However, patients are entitled to change their advance directives at any time. Such changes are often related to patients' experiences with illness in themselves or others. For example, some patients change their preferences in favor of more treatment during and after potentially life-threatening illness.[10]

Mr. Lang never gave much thought to being sick. He had worked hard, in all kinds of weather, wherever heavy construction was needed, since he was 18. Only recently had he begun to "run out of air." Now, at age 62, his doctors told him he had bronchitis and emphysema, and he had to stop working. He began volunteering at a hospital he had helped build the year before. He saw some patients on ventilators and decided that, no matter how bad his lungs got, he would never want to be kept alive if he couldn't breathe on his own. "When you get that bad, it's time to go." His doctor helped him complete an advance directive with this in mind.

That winter Mr. Lang caught a "flu" that wouldn't go away. He got progressively weaker and finally was unable to leave his bed. He was dizzy and had shaking chills. His neighbor called an ambulance, and he was taken to the nearest hospital, where he was found to be confused and dehydrated. Further evaluation revealed bilateral pneumonia and hypercapneic respiratory failure. He was intubated for three days and improved with hydration, antibiotics, and aggressive pulmonary toilet. Five days later he was discharged home to his apartment with new medications.

Once home, Mr. Lang reconsidered his advance directives. He hadn't understood that his lung condition could worsen so fast, or respond so quickly to treatment. He also changed his mind about ventilators. He was grateful that he was too sick to refuse the ventilator at the other hospital and that no one had known about his advance directive. "That machine saved my life." With his doctor's help, he changed his advance directive to include a trial of mechanical ventilation, if indicated, to be withdrawn after a week if his doctors judged that there was no improvement.

In the absence of written advance directives, surrogate decision-makers and physicians do a poor job of predicting what kinds of care patients would want.[11] Surrogates tend to overestimate, and physicians underestimate, patients' desire for life-sustaining treatment. Although a "values history" is a useful adjunct, advance directives are most stable over time, most predictable for surrogates, and most durable legally when they refer to specific treatments that the patient would want or not want in specific situations.[12,13]

The Patient Self-Determination Act of 1991 requires all health care facilities receiving federal funds to inform patients of their right to complete an advance directive and to create policies honoring these documents. Ideally, however, discussions about advance directives should take place in the outpatient setting, long before admission to a health care facility. Although most physicians and patients are aware of and agree with the concept of advance directives, only 15 to 20 percent of either group has actually completed the documents for themselves.[14,15] Multiple barriers to these conversations exist for both patients and physicians.

Barriers to Discussing Advance Directives for Patients

Perhaps the greatest patient barrier to communication about advance directives is the expectation that the physician will take the lead in raising the issue. Most studies suggest that patients favor discussing advance directives, even if they regard the topic as potentially upsetting, but expect the doctor to bring it up.

Some patients have difficulty understanding and completing advance directive documents without assistance. They may be unsure about the meanings of some words, or about how to obtain, interpret, sign, and store the documents. They often want to know if the documents can be changed once signed and if signing precludes treatment for an acute traumatic injury such as a car accident. Patients living near state borders may ask if their advance directive will be honored in adjacent states.

Patients may have difficulty assimilating information about diseases, treatments, and outcomes in ways that facilitate decision making about advance directives. They may be unprepared for the complexity and uncertainty of clinical medicine, or they may have difficulty integrating technical information from their doctors with their own personal experiences, expectations, and values.

For some patients, advance directives seem personally irrelevant. They may feel too young and healthy to consider advance directives important, or they may feel that their doctors and families will take care of such decisions when the time comes. Others, citing a strong respect for life, feel that care should never be limited under any circumstances. Occasionally, patients fear that discussing advance directives would upset and divide family members. Finally, some patients are distrustful of others, including family members, physicians, and health care institutions. They question the motivations of those who wish to limit care and are fearful that if they complete an advance directive, they will forfeit control of their care to others whom they cannot trust.

Barriers for Physicians

Little has been written about physician barriers to communication with patients about advance directives. Since physicians are no more likely than patients to have completed an advance directive, it seems likely that many of the issues outlined above also apply to physicians.

Despite evidence to the contrary, some physicians continue to worry that bringing up the topic of advance directives communicates pessimism or loss of hope, and that patients will react with anxiety, depression, or even suicide. In fact, research shows that the small percentage of patients who are upset by these conversations remain grateful for the chance to discuss them. Some physician discomfort about raising the issue may be related to the ambiguity of multiple roles as lifesaver and healer, neutral scientist, guide and counselor, or intimate confidante. Physicians may feel ethically or legally vulnerable when they perceive that these roles collide (for example, when desire to save lives conflicts with the perception that aggressive life-sustaining treatment may be futile).

In a study of resident physicians talking with patients about advance directives, the investigators observed three additional pitfalls.[16] First, they noted that insufficient technical knowledge about what the documents say and mean, and how to obtain and use them, were important communication barriers. Physicians were unprepared for questions about witnessing signatures on the documents, their applicability in acute traumatic injury, and where they should be kept. Second, physicians tended to use technical terms and jargon in describing both advance directives and life-support technology. They sometimes overloaded patients with too much information and missed cues from patients to slow down or clarify what had been said. Finally, they sometimes had difficulty eliciting patients' feelings and values. They made few explicitly empathic statements and few inquiries about what aspects of health and function patients felt it was important to preserve. Rather than viewing the session as an opportunity to initiate a dialogue about patients' experiences and values, or to hypothesize some specific situations and clarify patients' wishes, some physicians tried to reach premature closure on the issue by encouraging patients to simply sign the documents.

As a final barrier to discussions of advance directives, some physicians are pessimistic about how useful advance directives are in actually guiding patient care. They may question the stability of a patient's wishes over time, the ability of surrogates to accurately predict what the patient would want, and the practical "portability" of the documents across the multiple providers and facilities a patient may face. They may also feel that advance directives cannot adequately anticipate or guide decision making because of the complexity and unpredictability of clinical medicine.

Techniques to Facilitate Communication about Advance Directives

Several techniques can be useful in introducing the topic of advance directives to patients (Table 10.3). One is to place it in the context of routine office practice ("I tell all my patients about . . ."). Another is to place it in the context of preventive and collaborative care ("I know that you are particularly interested in learning about and planning for your own health care. Here is one way . . ."). A third is to take advantage of public or private events that raise the patient's consciousness about end-of-life issues ("You know, Congress passed a law recently that affects the health care of all Americans called the Patient Self-Determination Act. What it means is . . ."). For patients who may be reluctant or anxious about the topic, clarify your intentions with an announcement ("I'm going to talk about something now that many people don't like to think about, but I believe it's important . . ."). No matter how the topic is brought up, it must be accompanied by a disclaimer reassuring the patient that it is not a prelude to giving bad news ("Right now things are going well in your health and I have no reason to suspect that will change. However, we must always plan for the future and the possibility of unexpected events. One of the ways we can do this is . . ."). Letting patients know that you have completed advance directive documents for yourself may be reassuring to them and can be a powerful modeling device.

TABLE 10.3. Techniques for Discussing Advance Directives

1.	Bring up the topic yourself
2.	Explain that this is a routine procedure
3.	Answer questions about life-sustaining care
4.	Give information about advance directives forms
5.	Elicit patient's feelings and values
6.	Encourage an ongoing dialogue
7.	Help patients involve their families
8.	Provide resources and written materials

Several concepts are useful in discussing advance directives with patients once the topic is raised. The first is to try to strike a balance between giving information on one hand, and eliciting patients' values and feelings on the other. Here again, the best technique is to begin with some open-ended questions ("What sorts of thoughts do you have about these questions? How does it feel to be discussing these types of things?"). It is also helpful to find out if the patient has discussed his preferences with his loved ones ("Have you ever had the chance to talk this over with your spouse?").

When giving information, try to link it to patient questions or concerns ("What questions did your neighbor's condition make you think about for your own care?"). Remember to provide information in digestible "chunks," to avoid technical words and jargon, and to pause frequently to summarize and ask patients what they have understood you to say (Table 10.2). In describing diseases and treatments, most patients are less concerned with technical details and more concerned about outcomes of care, including expected functional status. In describing advance directives, it is likely that physicians will not know the answers to some technical questions. Help is available from many sources, including hospital patient advocates. Hospitals or concerned citizen groups often make available booklets that describe advance directives and answer specific questions. Patients can be encouraged to review these materials with their families prior to subsequent visits.

In eliciting patient feelings and values, begin by acknowledging that these conversations can be difficult but that many people have already given some thought to the topic. Express curiosity about the patient's values and the experiences upon which they are based. Try to identify not only what kinds of treatments or outcomes the patient desires, but also what he or she finds of most value (for example, the ability to speak or recognize loved ones). Recall that the goal of these conversations is to understand and respect the patient's wishes, not necessarily to limit treatment. For example, elderly patients may want treatments and accept qualities of life that would be rejected by many young physicians.

Some patients find that family members are reluctant to discuss advance directives or are divided on the issue. Reluctant spouses can be invited to a joint visit and encouraged to participate in the conversation. For the patient with a divided family (or, in the case of a gay couple, a lover versus a family), a person who thinks and believes as the patient does can be chosen to be a legal spokesperson. Patients who do not have a significant other to speak for them can often sign a directive to physicians limiting their care if they so desire.

The preliminary goal of bringing up and discussing advance directives is to initiate an ongoing dialogue, rather than to sign a document. Ultimately, though, specific decisions will have to be made if the advance directives are to be useful. Checklists describing specific treatment options and circumstances may be useful in helping patients to clarify and articulate their thinking and to eventually reach closure on these issues. The more specific the expressed wishes of the patient, the more likely they are to be legally protected. Many such checklists include an option for a trial of treatment which can be withdrawn after a specified period of time or if the physician's judgment is that it is unsuccessful.

Problem Areas in Discussing Advance Directives

Many physicians erroneously translate a completed advance directive document into an automatic "Do Not Resuscitate" (DNR) or "No Cardiopulmonary Resuscitation" (CPR) order in the patient's chart. In reality, however, the DNR order is written after the physician weighs the current medical circumstances with the patient's projected wishes and values as stated in the advance directive. If the likely outcome of resuscitation includes treatments the patient would not want (for example, prolonged mechanical ventilation, dialysis, or tube feeding), a DNR order should be written and discussed with the patient. However, the goal of most patients is to prevent futile life-sustaining treatment once the medical circumstances (diagnosis, prognosis, or short-term response to treatment) are known. These circumstances may or may not be clear at the time resuscitation is considered. Physicians may choose to inform patients of the futility of CPR with advancing age or multisystem disease. Physicians are not ethically obligated to provide futile treatments upon demand, but should inform patients of their judgment and explore the patient's goals and concerns. Patients often fear that a DNR order means that they will be ignored, abandoned, or denied other treatments.

Capacity to complete an advance directive has received little attention in the literature. Some patients with depression or dementia appear to be able to make choices about CPR that are as stable as those of nondepressed patients. Capacity to complete an advance directive is different than capacity to consent to treatment, and guidelines exist for eliciting and evaluating patients' understanding of advance directives.

CONCLUSION

Giving bad news and eliciting advance directives are important skills that are rarely taught to physicians. Sufficient medical literature now exists to formulate systematic approaches to both of these common clinical dilemmas. For both skills, an associated knowledge base, common barriers to communication, and techniques for giving information, providing emotional support, and eliciting patients' preferences for care have been identified. Physicians must tailor these approaches to their own individual styles and practices.

REFERENCES

1. Charlton, R. C., "Breaking Bad News," *Medical Journal of Australia*, 157:615–620, 1992.

2. Cassileth, B. R., R. V. Zupkis, K. Sutton-Smith, and V. March, "Information and Participation Preferences Among Cancer Patients," *Annals of Internal Medicine*, 92:832–836, 1980.

3. Krahn, G. I., A. Hallum, and C. Kime, "Are There Good Ways to Give Bad News?" *Pediatrics*, 91:578–592, 1993.

4. Sharp, M. C., R. P. Strauss, and S. C. Lorch, "Communicating Medical Bad News: Parents' Experiences and Preferences," *Journal of Pediatrics*, 121:539–546, 1992.

5. Billings, J. A., and J. D. Stoeckle, "Sharing Bad News." In *The Clinical Encounter: A Guide to the Medical Interview and Case Presentation.* Chicago: Year Book Medical Publishers, 1989. pp. 215–220.

6. Hogbin, B., and L. Fallowfield, "Getting it Taped: The 'Bad News' Consultation with Cancer Patients," *British Journal of Hospital Medicine*, 41:330–333, 1989.

7. Brewin, T. B., "Three Ways of Giving Bad News," *Lancet*, 337:1207–1209, 1991.

8. Links, M., and J. Kramer, "Breaking Bad News: Realistic versus Unrealistic Hopes," *Support Care Cancer*, 2:91–93, 1994.

9. Emanuel, L. L., E. J. Emanuel, J. D. Stoeckle, et al., "Advance Directives: Stability of Patients' Treatment Choices," *Archives of Internal Medicine*, 154:209–217, 1994.

10. Danis, M., "Stability of Choices About Life-Sustaining Treatments," *Annals of Internal Medicine*, 120:567–573, 1994.

11. Seckler, A. B., D. E. Meier, M. Mullvihill, and B. E. Cammer-Paris, "Substituted Judgement: How Accurate are Proxy Predictions?" *Annals of Internal Medicine*, 115:92–98, 1991.

12. Doukas, D. J., and L. B. McCulough, "The Values History: The Evaluation of the Patient's Values and Advance Directives," *Journal of Family Practice*, 32:145–153, 1991.

13. Emanuel, L., "The Health Care Directive: Learning How to Draft Advance Care Documents," *Journal of the American Geriatric Society*, 39:1221–1228, 1991.

14. Stelter, K. L., B. A. Elliott, and C. A. Bruno, "Living Will Completion in Older Adults," *Archives of Internal Medicine*, 152:954–959, 1992.

15. Brunetti, L. L., S. D. Carperos, and R. E. Westlund, "Physicians' Attitudes Towards Living Wills and Cardiopulmonary Resuscitation," *Journal of General Internal Medicine*, 6:323–329, 1991.

16. Gordon, G. H., and S. W. Tolle, "Discussing Life-Sustaining Treatment: A Teaching Program for Residents," *Archives of Internal Medicine*, 151:567–570, 1991.

RECOMMENDED READING

GIVING BAD NEWS

Annas, G. J., "Informed Consent, Cancer and Truth in Prognosis," *New England Journal of Medicine*, 330:223–225, 1994.

Buckman, R., *How to Break Bad News: A Guide for Health Care Professionals.* Toronto: University of Toronto Press, 1992.

Creagan, E. T., "How to Break Bad News—And Not Devastate the Patient," *Mayo Clinic Proceedings*, 69:1015–1017, 1994.

Fallowfield, L., "Giving Sad and Bad News," *Lancet*, 341:476–478. 1993.

Girgis, A., and Sanson-Fisher, R. W., "Breaking Bad News: Concensus Guidelines for Medical Practitioners," *Journal of Clinical Oncology*, 13:2449–2456, 1995.

Maguire, P., and A. Faulkner, "Communicate with Cancer Patients: Handling Bad News and Difficult Questions," *British Medical Journal*, 297:907–909, 1988.

Muller, J. H., and B. Desmond, "Ethical Dilemmas in a Cross-Cultural Context: A Chinese Example," *Western Journal of Medicine*, 157:323–327, 1992.

Quill, T. E., and P. Townsend, "Bad News: Delivery, Dialogue, Dilemmas," *Annals of Internal Medicine*, 151:463–468, 1991.

Reiser, S. J., "Words as Scalpels: Transmitting Evidence in the Clinical Dialogue," *Annals of Internal Medicine*, 92:837–842, 1980.

DISCUSSING ADVANCE DIRECTIVES

Danis, M., L. I. Southerland, J. M. Garrett, et al., "A Prospective Study of Advance Directives for Life-Sustaining Care," *New England Journal of Medicine*, 324:882–888, 1991.

Elder, N. C., F. D. Schneider, S. C. Sweig, et al., "Community Attitudes and Knowledge about Advance Care Directives," *Journal of the American Board of Family Practice*, 5:565–572, 1992.

Emanuel, L. L., "Advance Directives: What Have We Learned So Far?" *Journal of Clinical Ethics*, 4:8–16, 1993.

————., "Structured Advance Planning: Is It Finally Time for Physician Action and Reimbursement?" *Journal of the American Medical Association*, 274:501–503, 1995.

Emanuel, L. L., M. J. Barry, J. D. Stoeckle, et al., "Advance Directives for Medical Care: A Case for Greater Use," *New England Journal of Medicine*, 324:889–895, 1991.

Ganzini, L., M. A. Lee, R. T. Heintz, et al., "The Effect of Depression Treatment on Elderly Patients' Preferences for Life-Sustaining Medical Therapy," *American Journal of Psychiatry*, 151:1631–1636, 1994.

LaPuma, J., D. Orentlicher, and R. J. Moss, "Advance Directives on Admission: Clinical Implications and Analysis of the Patient Self-Determination Act of 1990," *Journal of the American Medical Association*, 266:402–405, 1991.

Silberfeld, M., C. Nash, and P. A. Singer, "Capacity to Complete an Advance Directive," *Journal of the American Geriatric Society*, 1141–1143, 1993.

INDEX